The Power of

Self-Care/Self Love:

A Physical Therapists Guide to Evolving
Into Your Higher Self

With love & health,

Jackie Castro-Cooper, MPT

Jackie Castro Cooper

i

JACKIE CASTRO-COOPER

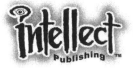

ISBN: 978-1-945190-92-6

www.IntellectPublishing.com

Cover Designer: Daria DiCieli
www.misschicnbeautiful.com

Intellect Publishing, LLC
6581 County Road 32; Suite 1195
Point Clear, Alabama 36564 USA
www.IntellectPublishing.com
Inquiries to: info@IntellectPublishing.com
First Edition

Important note: Readers are strongly cautioned and advised to consult with a physician or other licensed health care professional before utilizing any of the information in this book.

FV – 8

www.SelfCareSelfLoveBook.com

In Gratitude

I wish to thank my husband, Scott, and our children Alyssa, Logan, and Sofia, who have always supported and believed in me during the past decade of writing this book. I also want to thank John F. Barnes, Physical Therapist, who showed me how strong and capable I was to evolve into a more knowledgeable, loving, and generous being. I am grateful to Dr. Christiane Northrup who has created a path for women in the healthcare field by writing books that look beyond what has been laid before us, thereby transforming ourselves into more caring and loving beings.

Many thanks to Sarah Ban Breathnach for writing, *Simple Abundance,* which allowed me to evolve into each stanza of my life. I'm thankful for Oprah Winfrey's presence on my living room TV as she taught and introduced me to people who would help me become a better and healthier spiritual being.

Thank you to my editors: Maryann O'Gorman who took a global look and directed me into the style of this book, Author Johnnie Bernhard, who edited, mentored me, and kept me going, Nicole Langton for her good eye and for keeping everything in line to the bitter end, and Duke Sutherland who thankfully took on the difficult task of citing and re-editing over and over; he, too, kept me going. Terry Buchanan for guiding me early on and reminding me of the importance of empty ness, Marie Forleo for her life changing B-School, Risa Ladner for leading me in the right direction when I was stuck, and for Daria DiCielis' transformative divine book cover that represents all women. A special thank you to Betty Sue O'Brian, my natural physician, who also reviewed and edited and taught me many years ago to trust my instinct, be courageous, write well, and to open new ways of healing. Thank you for believing in me, Betty Sue!

Last, but certainly not least, a big thank you to the amazingly talented John O'Melveny Woods at Intellect Publishing for taking a chance on me and reminding me that all things are possible!

"Just when the caterpillar thought the world was over, she became a butterfly"

- Barbara Haines Howett

Foreword

Jackie Castro-Cooper, PT began learning Myofascial Release from me in 2006. She is a beautiful, intelligent woman of high integrity who has become one of my assistant instructors. It's a pleasure to have been part of her healing journey and now to watch her bloom. This book suggests, "Gently hold your hand and return you to your inner wisdom and your own ability to heal." Her personal stories and her own evolution's really do inspire and empower the reader to move forward and evolve. Judging herself and feeling unworthy held Jackie back for many years from becoming a physical therapist, but her determination and belief kept her going.

Using the proverb, You Are a House with Four Rooms, Jackie takes us into the physical, intellectual, emotional, and Spiritual rooms. She tells personal stories and then recommends healing methods that may prevent illnesses and heal you.

Not many authors that are not scientists or researchers talk about epigenetics, neuroplasticity, high vibrational frequencies, psychoneuroimmunology, and the hypothalamus, pituitary, adrenal axis, but Jackie explains these important topics with ease. She also discusses optimism, laughter, compassion, altruism, and gratitude and sites research that shows their healing effects on the body. In the four ways we can connect with emotions and heal Jackie encourages Myofascial Release along with journaling, yoga, and EFT, Emotional Freedom Technique.

This important book introduces the reader to not only healing modalities that will soon be mainstream, but also to the high vibrational frequency of love and the care that is needed to achieve it.

John F. Barnes, PT, LMT, is the President of the Myofascial Release Treatment Centers and International Myofascial Release Seminars. He is the author of, *Myofascial Release: Healing Ancient Wounds and Myofascial Release: The Search for Excellence.* John F. Barnes, PT has trained over 100,000 therapists and physicians in his highly successful Myofascial Release Approach®. He was named one of the most influential persons in the therapeutic profession in the last century in one of the leading therapeutic publications whose featured article was titled "Stars of the Century." In addition, John F. Barnes, PT has been a keynote speaker at the American Back Society Symposiums for over 25 years and presented Myofascial Release at their recent symposium whose theme was the most important advances in healthcare in the last century.

Dedication

I would like to dedicate this book to the first two women I watched care for and love themselves as they evolved; my grandmother, Carmen Maria Galindo, and my mother, Floralba Castro. They were fully connected to their divine bodies as they evolved through their years. They taught me: "Your body, mind, and spirit are Holy. Treat them as such," and "Joy comes only from you, who creates it."

This book is also dedicated to all my patients brave enough to stop the madness of an unfocused life to return their focus on health, growth, joy, and evolutionary metamorphosis. Regina Bonolo, and all the women on this earth, this is for you. The Self Care/Self Love movement has begun.

What calls one to write a book? My patients and participants in my presentations have all asked me to write a book. But for me, brace yourself. I'm going to say it, God. Yep the right side of the brain, Inner Wisdom, Source, Higher Self, Universe, Light, Holy Spirit, Intuition, or Inner Voice asked me to publish this book. When we connect or become one with the divine higher vibrational energy frequencies, wonderful things begin to happen. A paradigm shift occurs, a movement begins, a book is born. This book is a gift to all women to shift into their own ability to heal their ravaged hearts.

My heart was ravaged after I was born. Two weeks after my birth, my father left me. He left all of us, my mother and two older brothers, ages five and six. As a little girl I blamed myself for many years. I remember thinking to myself, "If I wasn't born, my mother would still have a husband and my brothers would still have a father." It wasn't until I was a teenager and my mom finally spoke about him that she said, "I was happy he left." I remember my heart healing in that very instant just like the Grinch, when his heart grew three sizes that day! I realized my birth allowed my mother to evolve, and I was meant to be here on this earth. My whole feeling about mySelf was different, I was free. I felt like I had been in a cocoon and hadn't even realized I was in one. This is the same for you. You are here for a reason but healing your ravaged heart must come first.

Women across the globe are suffering at an alarming rate: physically, emotionally, and spiritually. Self-Care/Self-Love are virtually nonexistent. Good news my friend! There are wonderful tools in here to help us heal and move forward. This book is a gathering of my life experience and knowledge of what has helped me, and my patients heal.

What makes me an expert to guide you on your evolving Self Care/Self Love journey? A Master's in Physical Therapy has opened a window to expand my mind and see the wonder of all possibilities of healing. When we dissected cadavers in the first semester of school, the intricacies, perfection, and specificity of the body were astounding to me. I remember saying, "How can this be? Every inch that I look at has a purpose! If everyone could unzip and open up their skin, they would definitely take better care of this perfectly designed miracle." I knew at that moment that our bodies, if treated with care and love, have a better chance of overcoming illness, healing themselves, and possibly preventing illnesses. What makes one a guide is one's own healing, evolutionary metamorphosis.

My early life as a dancer was purpose-driven and very exciting. Yet, it was filled with physical pain from falls and repetitive extreme use of my joints that lead to injuries, and emotional pain from constant rejections, audition after audition. Eating once or sometimes twice a day to keep thin disconnected me from my nutritional needs. The pendulum rebounded when the dancing stopped. I married and gained weight so quickly it stunned me. Becoming a personal trainer in New York City was the first awakening of my disconnect to my health. Giving birth to my first baby rendering me incapable of walking for three months, awakened me to the lack of care for new mothers. Then a master's degree in Physical Therapy educated me further to the disconnectedness from my body.

Beginning a practice in meditation and yoga integrated my body, mind, and spirit. The glue that connected everything was a thirteen-year journey studying John F. Barnes' Myofascial Release. The result was twelve years of my own holistic, integrative physical therapy practice, which has allowed me the honor of assisting my patients as they heal themselves.

This guidebook will introduce you to many simple tools that have changed my life. A wonderful author and editor said to me, "Write what you know." I am writing what I know, Johnnie Bernhard. Thank you!

JACKIE CASTRO-COOPER

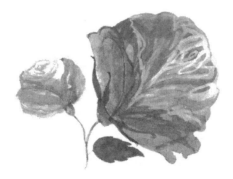

Table of Contents

Introduction

Your Health and Your Progressive Stanzas

There are many stanzas in our lives. A stanza is a group of lines set off by a space that usually has a set pattern of meter and rhyme. Our lives are the evolution of these stanzas and spaces all going through a metamorphosis, a coming out of a cocoon, revealing a masterpiece, YOU. Oh yeah. This earth has never seen the likes of you in all of humankind. Yes, beautiful friend. You are poetry in motion. Spread those wings!

There can be a sequence to our stanzas where we follow traditional patterns such as deciding whether to attend college, deciding whether or not to marry, to have children or not. Or nontraditional patterns may be followed, where there is no continuing education, but a job and career path. Whatever stanzas and spaces we use in the order that they occur is what defines each one of us uniquely. But hold on. The one priority we too often forget during the evolution of our stanzas is our health. Yes, how we treat ourselves and how we care and love ourselves is very important. They both play a vital role throughout each of the wonderful evolving stanzas of our lives.

"The events in our lives happen in a sequence in time, but in their significance to ourselves, they find their own order." --
Eudora Welty

The Power of Self Care-Self Love Book is written for women who are ready to accept the connection between their health and their progressive stanzas in life. As the United States charges ahead, we falter by having one of the least healthy female populations in the industrialized world. No matter our race, cultural background, or economic level, most of us are working too hard, caring for too many; we're financially depleted and seriously over stressed.

Spending time with awesome female patients in my physical therapy practice, I've noticed a common look on that first day of evaluation. As I lean across to shake their hands, our eyes meet, and I see pain, loss, and sorrow: pain from their inflamed physical bodies, loss from their disconnect to themselves, and sorrow from the realization that they don't know how they got there. While they were busy trying to make great achievements at work and in their personal lives, they completely cut themselves off from their health. It's as if they've been on auto pilot flying through severe turbulence for 5, 10, 15 years, and they come in limping and in a daze.

This is why I'm writing this book.

I want to tell every woman in the world that caring for yourself and loving yourself is what our grandmothers and great grandmothers did, and what we need to continue. Self-Care/Self Love for our intuitive, female ancestors was demonstrated in the physical work to grow and prepare food that would heal and sustain themselves and their families, their thoughts were on what was possible; they expressed their emotions to other women, and they believed in God or Gods. Today you can do the same, but you have more options.

This book gently holds your hand and returns you to your inner wisdom and your own ability to heal. The ability to heal, create, grow, and move forward will return. The words on these pages will bring awareness, evidence-based research, and real time answers on how to reconnect with the self through physical, intellectual, emotional, spiritual, and social choices. The goal of this guidebook is to inspire and empower women to care for and love themselves so they can evolve into the next stanza of their unique lives. How do I know about evolving and the vital importance of health? Simply put, I've lived these stanzas and am only halfway through, maybe? I think? Who knows??

The earliest memory I have of evolving was when I was five years young. I was in a ballet class and the teacher said, "Fly across the room like a butterfly." I immediately grew wings, became lighter, and felt as though wind was carrying me above the wooden floor. I remember the other little girls looked at themselves in the mirror. I didn't need to look; I could feel the transformation within me. Every cell of my body was feeling utter joy! I evolved into a dancer.

I was lucky to have a wonderful teacher, Sally Hammond, near my house. Her school of dance named after her, in Queens, New York, was my introduction to my first evolution. My love of dance blossomed, and at age fifteen, I joined the Windemere Ballet Theater. The world of dance was magical, but catastrophic on my body; I am still feeling the residual effects today. My life as a dancer was an unhealthy life. I treated my body as a machine, not a holy temple. The chapters in this book describe my personal experience, as I have evolved through my many stanzas and spaces, and how I've learned to heal.

As we'll see in Chapter One, Self-Care/Self-Love, I share a moment when I realize my body was trying to tell me something by ringing an alarm called burnout. I then present the top six health issues for women in the U.S. and introduce a method I use with my patients to increase awareness called "A House with Four Rooms."

In Chapter Two, The Physical Room, I describe what it felt like to lose my identity and evolve from one career into a "no" career or what Dr. Seuss calls, "The Waiting Place." I share my story of why I was unable to walk after giving birth. Then, I discuss the reasons why we need to physically move our bodies, as well as how to motivate ourselves to move. Lastly, I introduce you to something I've created for you called AST (Active Self Time).

Chapter Three, The Intellectual Room, shows you how to decrease a fever, and what the heck is epigenetics? I also discuss why optimism, gratitude, laughter, movies that make you laugh out loud, and brain cells help us heal.

Chapter Four opens the emotional door, and I share how my self-judgment and feeling of unworthiness prevented me from entering the career of physical therapy at an earlier age, why I went to Europe, why letting go of past traumas heals you, the four methods I use to heal myself, and the importance of choosing the right health care practitioner.

Chapter Five, The Spiritual Room, describes the connections between a visit with a cloistered nun, life force, collective consciousness--what scientists call the field--and high vibrational frequencies. We look at the effects of love and altruism on our health. To meditate or medicate, a new way to look at depression, the importance of nap time! Premenstrual truth and menopause. Science is great, but how can I apply it? And then a closing poem, "How I Began to Love Myself."

Chapter Six shows us the benefits of having friends and starts out with what I believe is one of the roots of pain, not belonging to a tribe. Then, we'll explore how the bonds of women and their stories can help maintain our marriages and how having a regular girls' night and the power of hugs can heal us. I'll give tips on healing an empty nest and how to apply healthy alternatives. Then I'll answer the question, Can relationship problems cause pain in your body? Science is great, but how can I apply it?

In Chapter Seven, I will show how evolving isn't easy through my personal story of not being good enough, and how believing in yourself and never giving up changes everything. Then, I share the four questions and go into the importance of creativity, especially if it's creating yourself. I then give you a simple worksheet I created to give my patients. This worksheet allows you to create your habit of Self-Care/Self-Love.

I conclude with a poem on how our deepest fear is that we are powerful beyond measure.

Dear friends, let's dive into the care and love that's been missing.

Jackie Astro Cooper

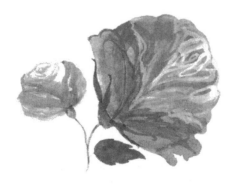

The Power of

Self-Care/Self Love:

A Physical Therapists Guide to Evolving Into Your Higher Self

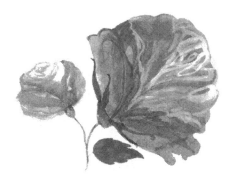

Chapter One:
Self-Care/Self-Love

What is Your Body Telling You?

One spring day, I was driving in my car during my last semester of the master's program of physical therapy school in Mobile, Alabama. Suddenly, I didn't know where I was. By that I mean, it felt like I was in a different town. I was disoriented and recognized nothing around me. I had never seen the buildings. The signs with the names of the roads were foreign to me. I didn't know where I had just come from or where I was going. Remembering how to drive was not a problem. I was just confused and couldn't make sense of my surroundings. I was scared and immediately began to pray. I grabbed my cell phone and called my husband, who was an hour away, to explain what was going on. He asked me the name of the streets where I was and then told me to pull over and breathe for a few minutes, and he would call me right back. His intention was to call my friends from school to come and get me back.

I pulled into a parking lot and right in front of me was a big sign with the name of a massage studio that unfortunately, I do not remember, or I would be publicly thanking her! I called my husband to let him know I was going to get a massage and would call him back in an hour. I got out of the car and sort of floated in as if sleepwalking. The woman greeted me and said she was about to close, to which I said, "I really need a massage because I feel very disoriented, and I'm in my last semester of PT school." She quickly escorted me into a beautiful room with heavenly music and began an hour of gentle, loving massage, spending a lot of time on my belly.

During that hour, I cried and felt like I was going back into my body. The massage therapist told me I was not sleeping enough, eating poorly, studying too much, and stressing out. I asked her why no one else seemed to be experiencing this, and she responded, "Who else has three small children, a husband, and is forty years old in your master's program?" I smiled and said, "No one." She smiled back and said in her beautiful Alabama accent, "Y'all burned out, honey. It's time to start taking care of yourself." That was my first experience with lack of Self-Care/Self-Love and burnout.

Burnout

In the early Seventies, Herbert Freudenberger coined the term "burnout." He was a child survivor of the Holocaust who later lived with an uncaring aunt who made him live in the attic. He ran away when he was a teenager and later became a successful psychologist in New York's Upper West Side. He worked twelve hours a day and then went to a bad part of town, the Bowery, to assist young people until 2:00 A.M. One day, his family was preparing to go on a vacation, but Herbert could not physically move from his bed. His analytical mind kicked in, and he began to wonder what was happening to him. It was not just exhaustion, and it was not just depression. Something new was occurring.

He decided to analyze himself and began speaking into a tape recorder for two hours. He then listened to his recordings. "I don't know how to have fun. I don't know how to be readily joyful." He remembered the drug addicts down on the Bowery with their blank looks and their cigarettes burning out. He wrote the book *Burnout: The High Cost of High Achievement*. Mr. Freudenberger said, "Burnout really is a response to stress. It's a response to frustration. It's a response to a demand that an individual may make upon himself in terms of a requirement for perfectionism or drive (King)." Are we demanding too much of ourselves?

From my experience the answer is yes, and it's the reason why I wrote this book. As women we are demanding too much from ourselves and seeking the unrealistic goal of perfection. I've been watching women drop like flies around me from an endless list of illnesses and addictions. I met a woman who once said she sleeps very little and is exhausted most of the time because she can't go to bed if the kitchen's dirty, or if the clothes haven't been washed. I understand the importance of keeping a house in order and clean, but do we have to sacrifice our health for it? Shouldn't we place our physical health before our other priorities? Can't we listen to our body as it screams exhaustion or illness in our heads and every cell?

We create burnout. Burnout stops us from seeing or feeling our declining health. How does our nation rank in terms of health? "Over the past ten years, only the U.S. has failed to make significant improvements in the probability of survival up to age fifty for women (Khazan)."

How can this be? I thought we were one of the healthiest nations in the world. The 2019 Bloomberg Global Health Index ranked the U.S. thirty-fifth healthiest nation out of 163 ntries (Miller & Lu). The World Health Organization ranked the U.S. at thirty-seventh in health systems out of 190 countries. Hmm, no wonder women and men are not making significant improvements. Come to think of it, the number of female patients between the ages of forty-five and sixty-five coming to see me is growing. In fact, in my patient load, that cohort is larger than the above-seventy age group. What can we do to change the statistics? What are we missing? We're missing Self- Care/Self-Love, my friends.

Most everything we do in our lives, work, family, and community, requires courage, commitment, balance, and stamina, but what does it cost us in health terms? Are we paying a high price physically for all our hard work? As you can see from the statistics, the answer appears to be heck, yeah! The top five health issues for women in the United States are heart disease, breast cancer, osteoporosis, depression, and autoimmune diseases. In 2016, lung cancer was added. These diseases are the high price women are paying in the U.S.

Are we also working so hard we don't recognize when our bodies are speaking to us? According to Dr. Saralyn Mark, senior medical advisor for the office on Women's Health at the U.S. Department of Health and Human Services, "You know what makes you feel good, you know when you don't feel well. Understanding your body is key (Mark)." She goes on to say that knowing our family medical history, educating ourselves, paying attention to our bodies, and taking charge of our health can help prevent ailments (Zamora). "Paying attention to our bodies" is extremely important. Pay attention to your body. I remember the first person I watched do this, my grandmother. When she was tired, she sat down. When she was sick, she did five things:

1. Drank a specific herbal tea for whatever ailment she "felt" to boost the immune system.

2. Gave herself an enema to remove toxins from the colon and allow better absorption of nutrition into the body.

3. Took a shot of a Colombian liquor called aguardiente, moonshine/firewater that can actually decrease coughing. Used in a hot toddy, it helps one sleep and feel better.

4. Prayed to God to heal her, and she believed it. *The body does as the mind believes.*

5. Went to bed early as sleep allows the immune system and the brain to work better.

I don't recall ever seeing my grandmother, or my mother, who worked outside the house, go to an extreme and "burnout." Together they raised three kids in a new country, learned a foreign language, supported a family of five on my mother's income and no dad to help. In this new millennium would our great grandmothers say we have devolved into unhealthy women?

When we disconnect from our body, mind, and spirit, we allow ourselves to be distracted. We shut down our intuitive, inner voice, the right side of our brain. We miss the opportunity to stop ourselves from burn out and "prevent" illnesses. Shouldn't we be asking ourselves, "How am I feeling?" "What do I need?" "What can I do to decrease my chances of becoming ill?" "What brings me joy?" "How can I prevent illness and keep feeling good?"

Prevention

Our medical system is not generally geared for prevention of illness. It's more focused on drugs that will destroy whatever is ailing us, oftentimes with side effects. What if the focus was on boosting our immune system and looking for the underlying causes of our symptoms, thereby preventing the illness from reoccurring? I believe this is what used to occur. My grandmother did it, we can too.

A hundred years ago, doctors came to the home and looked at patients *and* the conditions they were living in. They checked the color, temperature, and texture of skin from head to toe. They looked into the eyes, surveyed the tongue, smelled the breath, touched the abdomen and various other organs and parts of the body. They asked what foods patients were eating and what patients were drinking. Today's doctors are rushed for time, so a lot gets overlooked. In my physical therapy practice, I do what I was trained to do in school. I look at my patients from head to toe in their shorts and sports bras. A one-hour evaluation is standard.

I look at the whole person, assessing circulation, blue or red lower extremities, red, blue, and white blotchy hands, visible inflamed blue veins, red chest, redness in the face, size of pupils, colors and inflammation of the eyes, ribs protruding, abdominal distention, skeletal imbalances, jaw imbalances, inflamed/swollen areas, difficulty breathing; weakness, lack of sensation in the feet, etc. Nothing is overlooked. And patients notice.

Drug-induced Dementia

One day my patient came in and shared a frustration she was having. She said, "Can you believe my mom was diagnosed with drug-induced dementia?" I said, "What? How can that be?" She said her mom was never told the medications could cause her to lose her memory and act strangely. "We were supposed to read the label, look at the side effects, and know for ourselves."

So, now medications are causing dementia? I felt like a first grader learning a new bad word everybody else already knew. Everything changed for my practice from then on. Many new patients come in with a long list of medications, but not much awareness of the damaging side effects. I now ask all my patients to look at their prescribed and over-the-counter medications and Google them or just ask their pharmacist if a side effect is dementia or cognitive decline. (Let's also not forget that alcohol is a drug and causes dementia.)

Ask Your Doctor Questions

I strongly believe asking our doctors questions makes us participants in our own healing.

- Why do you think I have this ailment? What caused this? What's the alternative to taking these pills?

- Is there another medication I can take with fewer side effects? A more natural option?

- If I change my eating, can you retest my blood in three months to see if I can stop taking this medication?

- Is this a drug which may cause dementia, a low sex drive, or affect my organs?

These are all important questions which need to be addressed if we are to empower ourselves for true healing.

What about preventing the need for medications in the future? We must be honest with ourselves and realize our poor food choices, an inactive lifestyle, and addictions are making us sick.

According to ACTION, Active Coalition That Influences Outcomes in the Neighborhood, prevention is key:

"Increasing the focus on prevention in our communities will help improve America's health, quality of life, and prosperity. For example, seven out of ten deaths among Americans each year are from chronic diseases, such as cancer and heart disease, and almost one in two adults has at least one chronic illness, many of which are preventable. Racial and ethnic minority communities experience higher rates of obesity, cancer, diabetes, and AIDS. Children are also becoming increasingly vulnerable. Today, almost one in three children in our nation is overweight or obese which predisposes them to chronic disease, and the numbers are even higher in African-American and Hispanic communities (Prevention Program)."

Prevention Can be Looked at as Self-Care/Self-Love

My dear friend, the key to prevention is becoming more intuitive, more aware, and more Self-Caring/Self-Loving. There is a proverb, "Everyone is a house with four rooms, a Physical, an Intellectual, an Emotional, and a Spiritual room." For a house to be livable and not become stale we must air out each room every day. These rooms are easy to remember when we call them the P.I.E.S. Because we all love pie! A simple worksheet I created helps all my patients open each room daily. The last chapter has the worksheet, but before you look at it lets define each room.

Let's open each room and look inside for some ideas, concepts, research, and real-life choices. A key factor in prevention is to become aware when something is changing as we evolve, and that The Power of Self-Care/Self-Love is an integral part of our evolving.

Let's look at the four rooms of P.I.E.S from a caring and loving perspective.

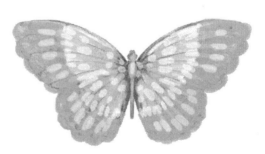

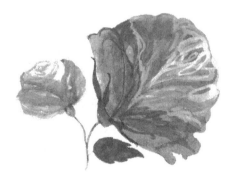

Chapter Two:
'P' The Physical Room
What You Do is Not Your Identity

When your body, mind, and spirit have been identifying with a career for a long time, and suddenly you stop that career, get ready for a roller coaster ride. In my case, my career, or I should say my life and what I thought was my identity, was dance. I was on file for *Cats* on Broadway with the casting agency Johnson-Liff for three years. While waiting for a life-changing phone call to be on Broadway, I did great work with equity and nonequity theaters all over the Eastern Coast of the U.S., Texas, and Mexico.

At age twenty-six, I asked God to get me on Broadway, get me an equity card, a union card that allows you to be hired by Broadway producers, or help me evolve. No phone calls, no Broadway shows, or equity card came for me that summer. Sadly, I let go of what I loved the most and said goodbye to all the beautiful nineteen-year young dancers lined up to audition behind me. I left the only world I thought I truly loved, the world of dance; the world where when your body moves, it creates all that is beautiful. A dancer is the artist's brush. What in the world was I going to do next? My identity was as a dancer, which is what I was "doing." I was not

13

prepared to evolve. I was not prepared for my life to change. The roller coaster ride was taking a nosedive, and I was not holding on.

This change in my life was so drastic I found myself crying, not sleeping, gaining weight, and eating more food than my body was accustomed to. Nope, not fruits and vegetables, but fantastic New York bagels and cheeseburgers were my cuisine of choice. I stopped taking all my dance classes. I stopped moving all together. I felt utterly lost and terrified. I no longer had a place in the world. I prayed. Deep inside God was guiding me to speak to someone who would listen, someone who would guide me through this space into my next stanza. I asked my friends for recommendations and realized almost everyone I knew in Manhattan was seeing a therapist. Needless to say, I had plenty to choose from.

I found a wonderful therapist, and on our first meeting she asked me, "Why are you seeking therapy?" The first words out of my mouth were, "I'm a dancer. I don't know how to be anything else." She responded, "You are confusing what you do with your identity. You are not a dancer, you are Jackie." The words she used were foreign to me. This was extremely confusing because my body, mind, and spirit were stuck. I felt like she was asking me to peel off my skin. You know when you must peel off a sticker from the backing and you can't find the edge? I couldn't peel myself off. There was no edge. I didn't know it, but I was in that space before my next stanza. I was a turtle on my back. The therapist recommended taking long walks in Central Park, going to the gym, meditating, reading inspirational books, doing things I loved, being with people I loved, and focusing on doing everything slowly and with great focus. She was teaching me how to reconnect with mySELF, which meant reconnecting with my body, accepting my new life, healing, and evolving.

14

Stubbornly, I told her I had no life and that I was nowhere. She had me buy *Oh the Places You'll Go* by Dr. Seuss. I felt silly asking for it in Barnes and Noble, but when they escorted me to the adult section, I was pleasantly surprised. I walked a lot that day, remembering her advice to physically move. I came home and sat down in a quiet place to read my new colorful children's book. The floodgates were opened! I cried and mourned the death of my life as a dancer, a label I gave myself for eleven years, or maybe even more, from that fateful day when I was five and grew those dancer wings. The roller coaster ride leveled out. My grip on the handlebars loosened. I sat back gently holding on. I knew right then where I was in my life. I was in the waiting place.

Dr. Seuss is so smart. I was in the cocoon preparing to be a newly evolved butterfly. I accepted where I was in my life, at a crossroads, the "space" between my stanzas. I let go of the handlebars. I slowly stepped out of the roller coaster. Off I went to do as I was told and joined a gym called Jack LaLanne. Remember him and his dog exercising on TV? If not, he is waiting for you on YouTube wearing his cute black onesie. I loved how he taught me as a little girl to move my body and become strong. More about Jack later in this chapter. For right now, do you know how many joints you have in your body and why?

We Were Divinely Designed to Move

The human body has over 300 joints, so we're divinely designed to physically move. As modern humans, homo sapiens, we've lived on this earth for about 300,000 years. Hunting, gathering, and using tools are what our bodies did to survive. Unfortunately, physical movement for those of us who live in industrialized nations today is becoming less and less important. People in both Europe and the U.S. are decreasing in physical activity. "Physical activity seems to be disappearing from life. People drive more – and further– than ever, work at increasingly sedentary jobs, and spend their leisure time on increasingly sedentary pastimes. Technological advances mean that even the simplest tasks are becoming mechanized, and people don't need to use as much energy to survive (Cavill, 2)."

When I was stuck in that difficult time in my life and couldn't let go of my identity as a dancer, I wasn't able to evolve into my next stanza because I didn't know who I was. I didn't know mySELF. I had lost what I thought was my identity. I was peeling off the label. I was shedding the "doing" in my life and connecting with the "being" in my life. I was moving my body as my therapist recommended. Opening the physical room was part of my healing.

I had experienced the death of what I thought was my own identity, but I was moving into the time space before my next stanza. Moving my joints out in nature helped me to revive mySELF. The self does not need a label. The self needs only to be in the NOW, in the present. Sensing and "being with" its own evolution. This is really hard to do if we're separating ourselves from what makes us feel alive, from feeling our heart pumping blood through our arteries and veins, and from inhaling and exhaling deeply into our lungs. It makes us feel alive to experience the sun on our skin or the smell of trees, the exhilaration of climbing to the top of a mountain, or the view of the expansive ocean, or to have the wind on our faces.

There will be times in our lives however, when it's physically impossible to move. This happened to me after the birth of our first child.

During pregnancy my body was evolving and changing drastically. By three months, I was wearing Scott's tee-shirts, and I gained weight rapidly. After six months, I started to have pain in the front of my pelvis. Each month I would tell my doctors, but they would say it was normal. But my intuition, God, was telling me something was wrong.

In my eighth month, I couldn't roll over in bed without excruciating pain in the same pelvic region. The doctors finally said, "Your baby's head is pressing on your pubic symphysis, that area is made of cartilage. Go get a maternity support belt." I bought the belt and it was helpful, but something told me I should've started wearing it back when my pain started. To make matters worse, I began early contractions, so I was put on bed rest. Of course, I gained more weight the last six weeks. The beautiful day finally arrived, and I gave birth to a 9.9lb baby girl. With the great joy of giving birth came the shock that I couldn't walk. My diagnosis was separation of the pubic symphysis.

Three nurses came into the room the next day determined to get me out of bed and walking. I told them, "I can't roll over because of severe pain, something is wrong." They encouraged me and said I could do it. While clenching my jaw and trying not to scream, I allowed them to help me sit up, then after a few minutes, to stand. Once I was standing, I knew the worst was about to happen, but I didn't care. I had to go home with my new baby. I tried to take a couple of steps, and when I did, I passed out from the pain. Now you know in the movies a medical professional always whips out smelling salts when someone passes out? One nurse did that, and it was like taking a whiff of ammonia to the power of ten! I can still smell it in my memory all these years later.

The three nurses carried me back to bed and called my doctor. There were no women's health physical therapists in the hospital, but the doctors wouldn't discharge me until I could walk with a walker. After a week, I held the walker and my upper body up and dragged my feet for four steps. I went home, and my neighbor, Powell Griggs, and my husband carried me up three flights of stairs to our New York City apartment in a chair. Who needs elevators? The next day I called my physical therapist for a referral to someone specializing in women's health, and he found Peggy Brill, PT. Three months with Peggy, and her love and compassion brought me back to life. Hence the reason why I'm a women's health physical therapist. During those ninety days, I learned how to breastfeed, eat organically, focus on my physical body, and connect with my own innate, God-given ability to heal. Thank you, Peggy for planting the seed in my head that I should write a book. It only took twenty-five years!

This was one of the most difficult times in my life, but all along I remembered what my grandmother, Carmen would say, "Through all of our pain and suffering we become stronger and more compassionate people."

Not having the ability to walk for anyone is terrifying, but for a former dancer it is a death sentence. If not for Peggy Brill and my family and friends connecting me to my own strength, it would have been a dark time. Around November 1994, towards the middle of my three months of physical therapy, I remember being able to walk, but not yet able to roll on my side to feed the baby. It was 4:00 A.M., and I sat in the rocking chair to nurse her and turned on the TV so I would not fall asleep. What was on TV? *Oprah*. The show was about courage and becoming the best you can be.

I believe in my heart that from then on, not only did I become a fan of Oprah, but I began to see that believing in myself and caring for *me* was the most important act of courage I could ever do for myself and my family. This changed everything. In my heart I knew I had evolved into a mother. As the flight attendant always says before takeoff, "place the oxygen mask on yourself before you place it on your child." This meant I had to slow down, care for myself, and delve into my new career, Motherhood. To be a good mom you must first mother yourself.

I wanted to stay home and raise my new baby, but you can't do that in New York City without two jobs. So, we moved to my husband's beautiful hometown of Biloxi, Mississippi, on the Gulf Coast. I evolved into a new place and physical movement was possible. I left New York City and all my family, friends, and coworkers. This allowed us the freedom to live on a single income and own our home. Unfortunately, I felt the familiar sensation of being at a crossroads, the "space" between my stanzas.

Biloxi was beautiful, but I was thirty-two with a new baby and extremely alone. I was indoors watching too much TV and still recovering from the fact that I couldn't walk very well after the pregnancy. I remember one day after I did my physical therapy exercises, I said, "Get out of the house and walk. Stop feeling sorry for yourself." I put my baby in the carriage and walked outside for forty-five minutes. It was exhilarating! I was connected to mySELF. Sure, everything was different. I felt alone, but I had the right to feel these emotions. I was experiencing a severe evolutionary change. I was a mom with no mother nearby, or friends from NY and now in the very warm South. Yet I knew, after that walk, it would be okay. I was living in the moment. I remembered to connect with mySELF.

19

Later, I went to a bookstore and saw a beautifully decorated book by Mary Engelbreit. When I opened it, the page read, "Bloom Where You Are Planted." The quote from St. Francis de Sales (1567-1622) struck me like a lightning bolt! I knew that if I was to thrive during my evolution, I needed to be physical and connect with my body, mind, and spirit, with mySELF. This allowed me to accept this new beautiful town in the South. I chose to learn more about the wonderful French and Spanish history of Biloxi, MS, since I was going to bloom here. I would learn to live without an Autumn, walk in ninety-five-degree weather, eat raw oysters, fried shrimp po-boys, and crawfish, although I'm still working on that last one! How do we motivate ourselves to move? Well, AST of course.

What are some ways we can introduce physical activity into portions of our day? How can we connect with the part of our DNA that needs to move and be active? Well, I have created AST, Active Self Time. I realized when I was raising my kids, I was a better mom and wife if I got away two to three times a week for forty-five minutes to two hours and did some physical activity.

One Saturday morning I blurted out the sentence, "Bye everybody. I'm going for some active self-time, and I'll be back in forty-five minutes." My husband knew I was going for a walk in the neighborhood, but he never heard me say those strange words, and our three kids had no idea why I was leaving the house without them. Before they could ask "What is active self-time?" "Why is mom leaving the house without us?" I was already out the door.

When I came back, everyone was watching TV, and to my amazement the kids were perfectly fine. I, however, had again felt that familiar heart pumping blood through my arteries and veins, and my lungs expanding and contracting like crazy! A huge weight had been lifted off of my slumped down, heavy shoulders. Immediately, I knew I had melded "me time" with "physical activity," and it was called Active Self Time, or AST!

Since then, I've been encouraging myself and all my patients to use the phrase, "Active Self Time," which is a little twist on "Me Time." Write your "AST" into your schedule. Sit down with your monthly calendar, and with a highlighter choose three times a week you will dedicate to moving or jumping for joy for ten to thirty minutes. If your calendar is on your phone, highlight accordingly.

Why is it better to do AST with joy? To paraphrase from an interview with P. Read Montague PHD Prof. of Neuroscience at Baylor College of Medicine, and Gregory Burns M.D. PHD Prof. of Psychiatry at Emory University from the documentary, *Happy;* Dopamine synapses die off after we are teenagers, but aerobic exercise done with "joy" decreases the rate at which these synapses die, therefore possibly preventing Parkinson's disease (Montague)." Many patients don't like the word exercise, so writing down AST and signing their initials usually seals that time for them. AST includes any movement which brings joy: walking, biking, hiking, swimming, kayaking, CrossFit, circuit training, Zumba, Pilates, yoga, jumping on a trampoline, or just putting on dance music and moving. Sorry, housework is not on the list!

Joining classes and creating new friendships with other women is very healing--more in Chapter Six. Nature heals you, so choosing an outdoor AST at least twice a week increases your sense of wellbeing, promotes vitamin D intake, and improves mood during AST.

My personal favorites are a yoga class, walking outdoors, Zumba, treadmill walking, and circuit training at the gym. But, if you're not into classes or gyms, there are lots of other options. These include self-motivating devices such as smartphones, watches, bracelets, and computers. Movement has never been easier. I dare you to pick one from this list:

<u>Smartphone apps</u>

Walking pacer app

My Fitness Pal app

Zumba Fitness app

Pilates app

Sport Me Running app

Simply Yoga app

Cyclemeter GPS app

Daily 7-minute workout app

Interval training, "Interval Timer HIIT" app

<u>Bracelets</u>

Fitbit

Bellabeat leaf

LETSCOM Fitness Tracker HR

<u>Computer</u>

YouTube videos

Yogaglo.com

DoYogaWithMe.com

yogainternational.com

gaia.com

Fabulous news! According to Edward R. Laskowski, M.D. from the Mayo clinic, "Even brief bouts of activity offer benefits. For instance, if you can't fit in one thirty-minute walk, try three ten-minute walks instead. What's most important is making regular physical activity part of your lifestyle (Laskowski)."

Thank you Dr. Laskowski. There is hope for all of us. Choose what will motivate you to move and just do it.

Now let me present my first mentor, Jack!

I grew up learning about healthy exercise with The Godfather of Fitness, Jack LaLanne. Jumping Jacks were named after him. Back then, we had no computers, no smart phones, smart watches, or bracelets, just Jack, so we had to stick him in here. Jack was that a FitBit on your wrist? He kept exercising until he died at the age of ninety-six. He was the first westerner to bring an awareness to the importance of 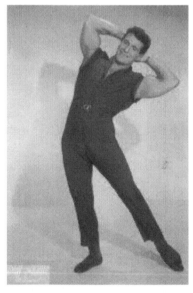 physical activity, the dangers of smoking, the benefits of eating fruits and vegetables, and working out with our dogs. ♡

According to the National Cancer Institute, regular physical activity also lowers the risk of breast and colon cancer. Although the research is not finished, endometrial and lung cancer also appear to be lowered with physical activity ("Physical").

Before we leave the physical room, I would like to mention something I found fascinating. Strength training increases our cognition--thinking, understanding, learning, and remembering--and may prevent dementia! I ask all my over-forty patients to start resistance training or lifting weights for thirty minutes three times a week (Chang).

Science is great, but how can I apply it?

When you identify yourself with the work that you do, it may be time to ask yourself if you're stuck or if you need to evolve. Remember, you are not your work. You are a Masterpiece all on your own. Get out of the house and walk, please. It will still be there when you get back, and the members of your family will be happy you left. Heck, you'll be happy you left. Choose Active Self Time, AST, that brings you joy, add it to your calendar, three times a week, and don't forget strength training!

This chapter has introduced the amazing benefits of physical activity. With hundreds of joints, we are divinely designed to physically move. If we combine physical activity with how we think and feel, it raises us to a new level of awareness.

The next chapter will introduce just how powerful beliefs and thoughts are and how they can affect your body and even your genes.

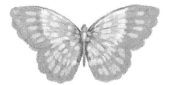

Chapter Three:
'I' The Intellectual Room

Beliefs and Thoughts

One day I came home from work with a fever. The thermometer read 102 degrees. My husband said, "I'm giving you two Tylenol." My response was, "Wait, I want to try out what John F. Barnes says to do and allow my body to glow with divine loving light and heal myself." My husband looked at me like I was crazy and said, "I'll be back in one hour to take your temperature again and give you the Tylenol." He had started to walk away when I said, "Wait I need a kiss and a hug so I can heal." He turned around and kissed me on the cheek. Husbands turn into chickens when there's a slight chance they can catch what they think is the plague.

I lay in bed and visualized my whole body glowing and repeated the phrase, "I am healing myself with my divine loving light, the Holy Spirit, and bringing down my fever." I remember going in and out of sleep. An hour later, my husband came back in, took my temperature and announced 100 degrees with the simple remark, "Good job," and walked away. That's it? This was a miracle! That night I gave myself permission to heal completely, and I broke into a sweat. The next day, I woke with no fever and felt great. I did it. It actually worked! I decreased my fever using my beliefs and thoughts. This miracle has a name, Epigenetics.

Let's dive into this little known, exciting field, which shows us how our beliefs and thoughts have a direct effect on our health.

Epigenetics

Dr. Bruce Lipton, author of, *The Biology of Belief; Unleashing the Power of Consciousness, Matter & Miracles,* tells us our thoughts and what we believe can change the environment of our cells/genes and therefore our health. This is actually a field of study called Epigenetics. The word means control above the level of the gene. After a few seconds of a thought our genes, located in our cells, receive the thought as a message through IEG's Immediate Early Genes. This thought message or energy changes the environment of our cells to do what they're told.

When I brought my own fever down, I did two things. First, I inwardly said, "I am healing myself with my divine loving light, Holy Spirit" and then I said specifically, "I am bringing down my fever." My belief was that I was doing it at that moment with divine light, Holy Spirit. My thought was to decrease my fever and heal. I didn't know it then, but according to Dr. Lipton my conscious mind (manual control) was telling my subconscious mind (auto pilot), which controls 95% of what occurs in our bodies, what to do. I was telling my 50 trillion cells what to do. My cells were banding together and following a "collective voice" a constructive belief. I could have also chosen to not believe and have a negative thought or destructive belief and the fever would not have gone down (Lipton, 176).

Since genes are inside of our cells, I was also sending a message to my genes to heal me. "Genes cannot turn themselves on or off...Something in the environment has to trigger gene activity. Genes do not control life (xxiv)."

Dr. Dawson Church, author of *The Genie in Your Genes,* agrees with Dr. Lipton. The environment that activates genes includes both the inner environment--the emotional, biochemical, mental, energetic, and spiritual landscape of the individual. And the outer environment which includes the social network and ecological systems such as food, toxins social rituals, predators and sexual cues affect gene expression (Church, 37).

The outer environment is our nutrition, toxins in our food, home, workplace, and neighborhood. The inner environment means our emotions, past traumas, how we feel about ourselves, how much we love ourselves, our stress levels, spiritual connection, friendships, family support, and what you believe can change. A good example is when Dr Lissa Rankin, author of *Mind Over Medicine, Scientific Proof That You Can Heal Yourself,* had an "Aha" moment after listening to Dr. Lipton explain, "When we see someone we love, the brain then releases oxytocin, dopamine, endorphins and other positive chemicals into the blood that is the environment of the cell. The blood changes the body's cell structure, and the cells change on a biological level. However, when we see someone as threatening, the brain releases stress hormones and other fear chemicals which damage the cells (Rankin, 28-29)." Damage our cells? Our thoughts and beliefs tell the brain exactly what chemicals to make that will hurt or heal us.

Now, let's look at the power of optimism and a new telenovela.

"Change the way you look at things and the things you look at change." --Dr. Wayne Dyer

Optimism

I believe one of the reasons I survived all of my evolutions thus far is because I was raised to be an optimist. The word was never uttered by my mother or grandmother, but it was understood. The following is a glimpse of my mom overcoming a difficult time in her life during a heart-wrenching moment resembling an episode of a soap opera or a telenovela.

My mother came to the U.S. from Bogota, Colombia, to escape an abusive, alcoholic, womanizer husband and raise her three children in freedom. Manhattan was where they spent their honeymoon; therefore, she instantly fell in love with the magic of New York City. I say magic because she was under its spell. She never felt more vibrant and alive. In her heart, she always knew she'd return to NYC one day and call it home.

Six years into their marriage, and two weeks after I arrived into the world, my father left. He had done this before, but this time he never returned. One of my father's girlfriends was also pregnant while I was in the womb. My mother knew now was her time. She had had enough. It was time to leave the oppressive marriage and the machismo Latin American country where she was raised. Her optimism and power started to grow. Her focus on the future became razor sharp. God was telling her to bust a move. It was time to evolve.

Unfortunately, the papers required to take her sons to New York needed to be signed by her husband. She dressed up, put some lipstick on, and went looking for him at her in-laws' house. They said he was not there, but she waited anyway. When he walked into the foyer, he was upset to find her there. She locked eyes with him and smiled. His guard went down. Must have been the lipstick. She let him know all was well with the kids, and that she did not need any money. Her visit was just to let him know she was planning a short trip with the boys to visit her sister in New York City. All she needed was his signature on the documents, so she could buy the tickets. He refused to sign the papers, but she never gave up. She continued to pester him day after day until he finally caved in and signed. He and his family got sick and tired of her constant requests. As Elizabeth Taylor would say, "Put on some lipstick and pull yourself together."

During the months of preparation, her friends realized she was really going. She was doing this! They became terrified and their fear brought out their pessimism. They started to say things like, "You'll never get a job." "You don't speak English." "You're not educated." "You won't have a man to help you." Finally, one friend cornered her and said, "What do you think you're gonna do for work in New York City?" My mother being the optimist she is--and to shut her friend up--just said the first thing that popped into her head, "I'll do embroidery work." Her friend was not expecting such a quick precise response, so she backed off. My friend, if you're going to be an optimist, you have to walk away with love from the people who are not open to your growth, your infinite possibilities, and your evolution.

My mom finally left Bogota, Colombia, with my two older brothers, ages five and six. Before she left, however, she threw out, donated, and burned everything she owned. She wanted no memory of her past. She describes it this way, "I wanted nothing to exist from my past. My past was dead forever. Everyone in my past was also dead to me. I left my pain and suffering. I entered my new life." Mama was evolving, and you better get out of her way!

Guess what her first job was? Yep, she got a job in an embroidery factory! She didn't even look for that specifically. It was just the first job opening which came to her. She didn't speak English, didn't have a man, was not educated, but she was now an embroiderer. The power of optimistic thoughts, optimistic talk, and visualization are so profound. Say it, own it. The universe, God is listening!

Meanwhile, back in the old country, I don't think it would be a good telenovela if we didn't go back, I was five months old, living with my grandmother, and we were supposed to join my mom as soon as she could gather enough money for our plane ticket. I say ticket because back then you sat your baby on your lap and prayed there would be no turbulence and so no flying babies. My mother's sister had gone to the U.S. before her, so Mom slept in my aunt's living room with my brothers.

My aunt didn't know I existed. My mom left this minor baby detail out, on purpose, because my aunt was judgmental and had hated my father since day one, when she advised my mom not to marry him. As soon as she found out about me, she told my mom to find another place to live when I arrived. My aunt's stabbing words to my mother were, "How could you be so stupid to have another child with that man after five years?! You have no common sense. You deserve everything that is coming to you."

It gives me great pain and brings tears to my eyes to type those words into this book. I guess I feel shame and horror at the lack of love and compassion for my mother, from her own sister! But I type them here because the truth is our closest relatives will sometimes be our worst enemies. Love and compassion aren't always flowing from our immediate family members, but don't let that stop you. Forgive them. That's what my mom did. She forgave her sister. Focus on the few who do support you. One or two of them are all you ever need. Luckily, my mom had her mother to support her in everything. Now guess who ended up being my aunt's POA and responsible for her care? The baby she didn't want in her house, me.

The one thing my mom did not have to worry about was me; or so she thought. Back to the old country. I was still in Bogota safe with grandma. Mawelita, was a name I created squishing the words "mama" and "abuelita", grandmother, together. All was well until the day a Western Union telegram arrived. At work, my mother received the telegram.

"YOUR HUSBAND HAS FOUND OUT THAT YOU ARE NOT COMING BACK **STOP.** HE TOOK THE BABY TO HIS MOTHER **STOP.** THEY WILL NOT GIVE HER BACK TO ME **STOP.** TELL ME WHAT I SHOULD DO **STOP.** Your mother, Carmen."

When my mom didn't come back from New York like she said she would, my dad freaked out. He was so angry that my mom lied to him, he went to my grandma's house and just ripped me from my Mawelita's arms. Looking down at this telegram in her hands, my mom said she felt like she was having an out of body experience. This couldn't be happening. She felt like she was going crazy. The words in Spanish are, "Me iba poniendo loca." Her heart was pounding so hard she could barely breathe. She knew she had to run and be in the only place of refuge she could think of. On her lunch hour, she ran to the nearest church. As she ran, she could feel her heart tearing apart and drowning in fear. Through her flood of tears, she could see the church up ahead. The Church of the Holy Innocents in the garment district was and still is on 128 West 37th street on Broadway in Manhattan. The tall, gold-painted, gothic revival doors were wide open. Back then people didn't steal from churches, so doors were open all day.

She rushed in and fell on her knees in front of the altar. She blessed herself, put her hands together in prayer, and through what little breath she had, she said these words, "My Lord, (Dios Mio) I will do anything you want, anything at all. But please give me back my daughter. I offer you my right arm for her. I cannot live without her." It appears that back then, body parts were common offerings. She then lit a candle at the feet of the statue of St. Anthony, the patron saint of lost items and lost people. Mom's devotion and faith to the Virgin Mary and St. Anthony gave her a reason to not give up hope. She was optimistic. She placed it in God's hands. She BELIEVED God had a plan. She began to pray the rosary, which she knew Mawelita was doing at that very moment. Not knowing how to respond to the telegram, she just went home, held her boys in her arms, kept saying the rosary, and waited for God to tell her what to do.

The very next day another telegram arrived, "URGENT, YOUR MOTHER IN-LAW HAS DIED OF A HEART ATTACK **STOP.** PLEASE SEND TICKETS IMMEDIATELY FOR YOUR DAUGHTER AND I TO FLY TO NYC **STOP.** Your mother, Carmen."

I told you this was like a telenovela! My mother freaked out and thought she had killed her mother-in-law, but after a week she got over it. It turned out my father's grief was out of control, so he was in no shape to care for a baby. I believe he also felt it was God punishing him for the pain he caused my mother and bringing a new baby to his mom to raise didn't make her very optimistic. I know if my son ever brings me his baby which he stole from its mother to raise, I am not going to be happy, much less optimistic.

As of the writing of this book, my mother still has a two-foot statue of St. Anthony in her living room and prays the rosary every morning. She is a great example of evolving into her higher self. I can't say her age, but she says she feels around twenty-one. So, you may ask, what are the actual benefits of optimism?

The Benefits of Optimism

A 2013 study from the Harvard School of Public Health published in the *American Journal of Cardiology* says that, "Middle-aged participants who scored as optimists had higher good cholesterol (Boehm)." Upbeat thoughts have a positive effect on physical recovery from an immediate stressor.

A Dutch study started in 1985, classed a group of men as optimists and were found to be 55% less likely to have a heart attack or stroke by 2000. In the article, *Optimists have less heart risk,* it discusses their findings, "Optimists seem less likely to die of heart disease or stroke than pessimistic people. The Delfland Institute of Mental Health study of 545 men found the most optimistic were about half as likely to die from cardiovascular disease (Optimists)."

Positive thoughts also create a stronger immune system. Positive self-talk improves problem-solving during times of stress. Optimism and longevity have been linked after a 2012 study done by Dr. Nir Barzilai found that 243 centenarians had the qualities of a positive attitude towards life (6 Personality Traits).

Laughter

Did you know laughing, even if you fake it, is scientifically proven to improve your health? An incredible story of the healing power of laughter is the story of Mr. Norman Cousins. In the Seventies, Mr. Cousins was a political analyst who was diagnosed with an incurable spinal disease. He experienced pain twenty-four hours a day. One morning, he woke up and realized he had slept for about two hours without pain. He began to wonder why, and the only difference was that he watched a funny show the night before and laughed a lot. He decided to do it again, but for a longer time and to his surprise he had no pain during four hours of sleep. He began increasing his laughter time by watching comedy shows and funny films. He learned that ten minutes of laughing out loud was equal to two hours of pain-free sleep.

Mr. Cousins continued laughing more and more until he completely healed himself from the incurable disease! He wrote an article about his miraculous laughter healing, and it was published in the *New England Journal of Medicine* (Cousins). He published his book in 1979, *Anatomy of An Illness*. It was later made into a movie.

Dr. Joe Dispenza comments on Mr. Cousins' power of laughter, "Although scientists at the time didn't have a way to understand or explain such a miraculous recovery, research now tells us it's likely that epigenetic processes were at work. Cousin's shift of attitude changed his body chemistry, which altered his internal state, enabling him to program new genes in new ways (Dispenza, 35)."

Laughter was first formally studied for its healing effects in 1964 when Dr. William Fry, a Professor of Psychology at Stanford University, acquired the funding. He became the first Gelotologist, a laughter expert (Gendry). I had no idea this was a field of study.

Laughter has been studied and found to:

- Decrease stress hormones cortisol and adrenaline
- Improve the immune system
- Decrease blood pressure
- Increase beneficial tumor and disease killing cells
- Reduce pain
- Increase oxygen
- Massage internal organs
- Boost endorphins
- Burn calories
- Decrease health care costs by twenty-three percent

Laughter clubs were started by Psychologist Steve Wilson, and one can become a certified laughter leader with the World Laughter Tour! There are more than 16,000 laughter clubs in seventy-two countries. These groups can be found in corporations, police organizations, prisons, blind support groups, deaf and mute groups, neighborhood groups, and cancer treatment centers, where the original Dr. Patch Adams created therapeutic laughter clowns (Laughter Clubs).

In 1995, Dr. Madan Kataria and his wife created, "Laughter Yoga (Laughter Yoga)." Sebastien Gendry took laughter yoga to the rest of the world and created the, "Laughter Wellness Method." Mari Cruz Garcia created, "Conscious Laughter" and trains laughter therapists in Spain (Bienvenid@s).

At the University of Maryland, scientists found that laughter is good for the heart because it dilates the lining of blood vessels, which improves blood flow (University of Maryland).

A wonderful Chilean woman, named Ana, told me to wake up in the morning and stand in front of the mirror with a glass of water, smile, and laugh at myself. It works. It not only makes me laugh, as I look funny with my bed head hair, but I drink my water right away. I placed a little sign saying "laugh" on my bathroom counter as a gentle reminder. It's pretty hard to take yourself seriously after you laugh at yourself before you've had your cup of coffee or tea.

Here are movie suggestions that come from my in-depth scientific research on my Facebook group page :) Pop some fresh popcorn on your stove and sit down and laugh. Don't know how to make fresh popcorn? Put oil in a large pot just enough to cover the bottom and popcorn kernels two fill two thirds of the bottom in one layer. Cover and put heat to medium. When the first kernel starts to pop begin to move the pot around every six seconds until you hear the popping start to slow down. When you hear two to three pops, move the pot to a cooler spot on the stove. When nothing is popping, slowly remove the cover because the popcorn may still pop. Pour into a large bowl and enjoy.

Movies that make people laugh out loud:

Some Like It Hot The Jerk, All of Me, Father of the Bride, Fun with Dick and Jane, Liar Liar, The Proposal, Hollywood Nights, The Princess Bride, Oh Brother Where Art Thou, Trains, Planes and Automobiles, Ghostbusters, Bird Cage, My Cousin Vinny, City Slickers, Home Alone, Talladega Nights, Rat Race, Step Brothers, Austin Powers, Young Frankenstein, What About Bob, Blues Brothers, Pitch

Perfect, The Big Lebowski, Pink Panther-- A Shot in The Dark, Blazing Saddles, Anchorman, Monty Python, Beetlejuice, White Chicks, My Big Fat Greek Wedding, Bridesmaids

Comedians: *Gabriel Iglesias, Sebastian Maniscalco, George Carlin, Chris Rock, Adam Sandler, Dave Chapelle, Wanda Sykes, Ellen DeGeneres, Amy Schumer.*

TV series: reruns of *Friends, The Office, Seinfeld, The Carol Burnett Show*, and *America's Funniest Home Videos*

My all-time favorite YouTube video, *"Quadruplet Babies Laughing" (Quadruple).*

An easy way to stay optimistic and happy is to be grateful.

"If the Only Prayer We Ever Say is, 'Thank you' That Will be Enough." - Meister Eckhart

Gratitude

I started a gratitude journal in 1997, when Oprah mentioned it on her show. I was a stay-at-home-mom of two kids, a three-year old and a one-year-old. It was just a little experiment I was doing to see if it would actually make my life more peaceful. I don't remember why, but after a while I just stopped writing in my journal from 2011-2013, maybe because by then we had three kids. It was during this time that I felt disconnected from a sense of peace. My oldest daughter was going through a difficult time and our expenses were off the charts. When our kids experience difficulties, we need to be calm and ready. We can be easily triggered during times of stress. I was not calm, and often responded too quickly which is what usually happens when all hell breaks loose. I re-evaluated my life and found that what had changed was that darn gratitude journal. I was much calmer and more grounded when I wrote in my journal. It worked and I didn't know it. I began again to write five things I was grateful for every night before bed. The change was dramatic for me and for my daughter. I was less judgmental and became more of a listener. When you want to change others, it's you that has to change. Just to double it up, I now say the five (or more) things that I am grateful for while my husband and I pray together before we sleep. It's fabulous for our sleep and our marriage.

When we consider all we already have, our energy becomes less focused on what we think we lack; our glass does become half full instead of half empty. Heck, some days we're lucky we even have a glass. When we remember to be grateful, our lives become fuller. We have fewer wants, and we focus more on what we need. Do you have what you need? Do you have a place to live? Do you have food? Do you have a warm dry bed to lay your head on at night? Do you have clothes to wear?

Benedictine Monk, Brother David Steindl-Rast, author of *Gratefulness; The Heart of Prayer*, talks about not just gratitude, but grateful living. In an interview with Oprah on Super Soul Sunday he said, "Look all around you and see all you already have." He says happiness that lasts is called joy. The key to happiness is to trust life. If you trust life, you will be surprised with good things (Benedictine Monk). This is faith.

* * * *

An example of when I was not trusting life was when my husband, Scott, wanted us to be fruitful and multiply. One evening, Scott and I were sitting on the couch; we only had one evening off together with my two jobs, personal trainer and concierge. He asked me if maybe there was something missing in our lives? I said, "Nope." He said, "Don't you think it's a little too quiet? Maybe we need the sound of pitter-patter in our apartment?" I looked at him, shocked, and said, "We have two cats; there is plenty of pitter-patter in this apartment." Was this really happening? I never saw myself as a mother of a human, only cats.

Mothers are completely devoted to their children. I was completely devoted to ME. I looked at my husband. His face was filled with joy. He wore a big grin. He asked me to think about it. I told him I had to pray about it, write in my journal, talk to my "finally healthy" body about it, and would give him a response in a week. The first part of the week was horrible, my journal writings were filled with, "How dare he ask me to be a mom." "It's easy for him to say, 'Let's have a baby.' He doesn't have to pop one out." "I'm not good enough to be a mom. I'm too selfish." But as the days passed the words in my journal changed. My heart softened. At age thirty, I was removing the fear of becoming a mother. I was evolving again.

The night I was to give him my response was the night of the Concierge Ball at the Rainbow Room. I had on a long beautiful black dress, and Scott was in his tuxedo. We were slow dancing to an eighteen-piece orchestra, and he asked me if I had time to think about his question. I looked away and said yes, I prayed every day. I didn't think I was mother material. I didn't want our lives to change. I was happy where I was. I looked back into his eyes and said, "Unfortunately, Scott I must tell you . . . Yes, I would love to have a child with you." He was so confused. We took a picture at that moment in time, because I knew this was the biggest decision I would make in my life. This was a defining, evolving moment and one I will be eternally grateful for.

As life would have it, and as my mom always said, "Nothing worthwhile is easy." I thought I'd get pregnant right away, but that wasn't the case. So, I started a stricter, healthier regimen of eating, sleeping, exercising, meditating, writing in my journal, and having more fun. I just focused on the now and spent more time with my family and friends. I was still working two jobs, personal trainer by day, 6:00 A.M.- 2:00 P.M., and concierge by night, 4:00 P.M.- 11:00 P.M.

We moved from Manhattan to Astoria, Queens, for a more affordable apartment. We paid off debts and started saving to buy a home. After a year of trying to get pregnant, I remember writing, "God, what the h---- was the point of removing my fear and evolving if I'm not going to be a mom?" For the first time, there was no answer. That really confused me. My mom told me to stop trying and to let go and let God. Years later I would learn this again from John F. Barnes, who suggests letting go of the outcome and simply trust.

So, I did. I stopped trying to get pregnant and controlling my life. I accepted that I would not be a mother. But I needed a break. I left for a five-day trip to Marco Island to get away and accept my fate. I needed to trust God's path for me. And as soon as I did that, we became pregnant. It was the greatest gift at age thirty-one!

A final thought from Brother David Steindl-Rast. If we choose fear, we are not trusting life. The root of violence is fearfulness and the feeling of not enough. Be grateful for everything. After gratitude, another way our beliefs and thoughts are vital to our health is by waking up our sleeping brain cells.

Waking Dormant Neurons

Do we have the ability to wake up sleeping brain cells or neurons? Yes, we do. The first one who did this, that we know of, was a nun. In 1986, a researcher wanted to study the causes and prevention of Alzheimer's. Unfortunately, the only way to do this then, and to truly know if someone had the disease, was by opening the skull and looking at the brain for plaques and tangles. Dr. David Snowden came up with a way to study a large group of women with similar backgrounds who did not smoke or drink and had updated health records. They were also close in age. He began his search for a retirement convent. The only thing he had to do was get the nuns to donate their brains after they died.

Dr. Snowden found 300 nuns from The School Sisters of Notre Dame in Mankato, Minnesota. They agreed to donate their brains to the pilot study after they died. The sisters' directive is to pray, learn, and educate, so it was easy for them to agree (Snowdon). That's when the largest Alzheimer's study began and continues today. Dr. Snowden asked all the nuns to keep a journal of what they had done before they retired to live in the convent and what they were doing now. Here is an excerpt from the article,

"In Mankato, Minnesota, in 1991, David Snowden sat across from a 100-year-old nun named Sister Mary, administering a test. He asked her to remember a list of words, to draw geometric shapes, and she passed each exam while she talked and laughed, constantly aware.

After Sister Mary's death at 102, a lab examined her brain. She had been alert and without memory loss, but instead of looking at a healthy brain, scientists saw one riddled with visible knots of protein—an indication of full-blown Alzheimer's disease. Sister Mary had the disease, yet she never showed any signs or symptoms of it! Sister Mary was part of a new research project on Alzheimer's called the Nun Study, and its findings not only shed light on the disease but inspired the largest Alzheimer's studies that exist today." I remember the day I read this article for my psychology class in 1997. I called my mom and with a high excited voice I said, "Mom, you are not going to believe this, but you can prevent Alzheimer's." I told her about Sr. Mary, and she loves nuns just as much as I do, so she started working out five days a week and till today she has not stopped. She already has a positive attitude and laughs a lot.

Sister Mary learned and did new things after she retired. She also sat and used a pedal bike for exercise. The nun study shows how our brains can heal us and prevent deterioration through plasticity, the extraordinary ability of the brain to modify its own structure and function. Believe you can learn something new and wake up dormant neurons. Living in a supportive community and having a deep religious faith can also prevent heart disease and stroke.

Neurologist Dr. David Bennett, who leads the religious order study wrote, "The brain reserve is basically its plasticity. . .. The ability to take a piece of the brain and fundamentally teach it to do something else. Our own ability to be flexible in understanding Alzheimer's is, it turns out, as important as the adaptability of our brains. While our understanding of Alzheimer's is still evolving, one thing is certain: even from beyond the grave, the sisters of the Nun Study still have a lot of teaching to do (Zarrelli)."

Another neurologist, Dr. Fotuhi recommends these lifestyle changes may help protect the brain as you age:

1. Decrease your risk of heart disease.
2. Do aerobic exercise to grow the volume of certain brain regions which tend to shrink during aging.
3. Learn new things--writing, and reading have been linked to better cognitive health in old age.
4. Being social is associated with higher levels of cognition. Loneliness conversely is associated with poorer brain health.
5. Laugh--depression in middle age is linked to twice the risk of cognitive decline.
6. Sleep well--Studies have found a relationship between poor sleep and risk of cognitive decline and Alzheimer's (Oaklander).

Today, doctors diagnose the disease with ninety percent accuracy by doing a physical exam, studying patient history, lab tests, and testing using neuropsychology. However, I just want to chime in and remind you that you don't have to own the diagnosis. Let go of the diagnosis. Heck let go of any diagnosis. Channel Sr. Mary and smile, be happy, learn something new, increase your exercise and evolve into a joy-filled life.

Science is Great, But How Can I Apply it?

What are your beliefs and thoughts lately? Are they stuck on a negative occurrence or are they optimistic? We have 50 trillion cells in our body, and they are ready to respond and heal your body depending on what you are thinking and feeling. You CAN heal yourself. Epigenetics shows you how. Remove your fear and discover the benefits of being optimistic. Laugh out loud and heal yourself. The only thing you have to lose is your pain. What are you grateful for? Do you always focus on what you don't have instead of being grateful and appreciating what you already have? Write down

10 things to be grateful for this minute. Notice how you feel? Wake up your sleeping brain cells, neurons, by doing something new. Be like Sr. Mary and prevent yourself from experiencing signs of Alzheimer's. Why not?

Changing our beliefs, thoughts, and words can bring us into a state of rest, triggering the parasympathetic nervous system. However, what if we dig deeper? What if we investigate the possible causes of our beliefs and thoughts? Would going into the emotional room allow us to become more optimistic, happier, more grateful, and healthier beings?

Yes, indeed.

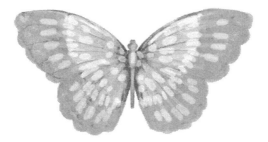

Chapter Four:
'E' The Emotional Room

We Must Heal our Past in Order to Evolve

"Whoa, I am not goin' in there!" The emotional room is not a popular room to go into. In fact, this room usually remains closed and locked. I grew up in New York City, so double locked. One deadly emotion is self-judgment. Judging ourselves is a hammer we pull out and use on our head way too often, think Three Stooges.

Self-Judgment

Have you ever heard someone say, "You are your own worst enemy"? Those words are sadly true. At the age of nineteen, I had one of my first experiences with self-judgment. As a dancer, I twisted my ankle many times and was sent to a physical therapist, Abby Corsun Symms. I'd never met a physical therapist before. Her demeanor was comforting, patient, and caring. She was so smart. She was an angel. She knew everything. She made me feel I could dance again. She told me, "You're going to be alright. You will heal." Anything I asked her, she had an answer for. Something inside of me sparked like a firecracker. I wanted to be like her, a physical therapist. For that one moment in time, I felt myself reaching for something new. Something other than dance. Something which I knew was ME! I felt my physical therapy wings peeking out, but something stopped them. With my next breath I could feel the spark of the firecracker just fizzle out. I could feel the twinkle and excitement in my eyes darken. I told myself something I had never said before, I wasn't smart enough and I wasn't good enough. I can feel it right now in every cell of my body. Abby was holding my swollen, painful ankle, and my body started to curve inwardly. I can feel that lack of confidence and unworthiness right now. It brings me to tears still to this day. I cut my own PT wings. Heck, I didn't even let them come out long enough to cut them. I used the excuse, "I hate school. It will take forever." Instead, I continued following my dream of becoming a professional ballerina.

A ballerina's life looks pretty and easy on the outside, but it's hard as hell. I was an unhealthy eater and followed what all the other dancers did in the Eighties, focused on being very thin. I fell more in love with ballet, but according to my mom, I had to keep going to college. No one had graduated from college in my family, so my mother reminded me, "You can follow your dream to be a dancer, but you will finish college. You will be the first one."

Queens College was not close, but it had great professors and a beautiful campus. On a typical day I had one meal to stay thin, college classes from 8 A.M.-12 P.M., dance classes in the afternoon in Manhattan, more dance classes and rehearsals at night. I worked in a French pastry shop on the weekends. My life was busy. No focus on health. I graduated from Queens College with a political science degree, because originally, I thought I would pursue law. Back then, not many dancers went to college, so it was a big accomplishment for me. My thoughts began to wander, and I found myself feeling like I wanted to visit Europe for a while.

I left home at the age of twenty-two, just me and a backpack, and headed to five European countries where I fell in love with local fresh food and auditioned for several ballet companies. Europe was magnificent, but not easy. The audition period for ballet companies is always in January, so I experienced lots of snow and freezing temperatures.

Food was a joy in Europe. Belgium was the first country I visited. I will never forget eating at a beautiful restaurant in Brussels, in the city's popular square. As I walked in, people stared at me. I had very long black hair, a long black coat, black winter boots, an enormous black backpack, olive Colombian skin, and I immediately locked eyes with an older gentleman waiter.

This wonderful waiter escorted me to a pretty table next to the window, with a candle and flowers. I had a view of the square and I was grateful. He walked away to bring a menu, and I quickly took out my Belgian handbook. It said I could speak French or Dutch in Brussels. I chose French since I had learned it in high school. The menu was not easy to read, so I basically just looked at him and said, "S'il vous plait, commander pour moi," please order for me. He appeared very excited and started to speak to me in French, to which I responded, "Parlez-vous Anglais? This was confusing to him. Apparently, he had never seen a long dark-haired Colombian who could speak a little French but preferred English. He spoke in English with a puzzled look on his face, "Where are you from?" I told him. He was confused and said, "I thought you were Turkish."

An exchange between two strangers from different worlds lasted two and a half hours. He couldn't believe I had traveled by myself in the dead of winter to audition for multiple ballet companies in five countries. I couldn't believe he had been a waiter for thirty years. It is a well-respected career in Europe. He ordered me some type of meat, potatoes, and Brussels sprouts. He almost choked when I announced that I had never eaten Brussels sprouts. The whole meal was sublime, and I fell in love with sprouts and my old-enough-to-be-my-dad waiter. We discussed many things: People don't need to eat in their cars when they allow time to have a good lunch. Fresh fruit and vegetables should always be the largest portions of a meal, and fresh flowers should be on the table. Meals shouldn't be rushed; they should be experienced. I learned to eat well for the first time.

I landed one job offer in Charleroi, Belgium, but I would have had to stay for two months and work for free until I received my work visa. That was a big no for me, so I continued on to Switzerland, Germany, Italy, and France. I stayed in hostels as the snow increased and temperatures dropped. Auditions were brutal, and loneliness crept into my heart. My confidence waned, and I began to lose interest in doing my best during auditions. My self-judgment grew stronger, "Who do you think you are coming here to these countries not even speaking the language? Everyone dances better than you. Everyone is even prettier than you." My dream and interest in living abroad as a ballerina faded. The hammer of self-judgment was too strong, and my home sickness was overpowering. I decided to go back to New York to evolve into musical theater. I dreamed of being on Broadway.

We all judge ourselves to some extent. These thoughts and beliefs, as we saw in the previous chapter, have a biochemical effect. The following words are so powerful they might as well be a door slammed in our face: "I am not good enough, smart enough, pretty enough, or strong enough. I am a failure."

According to an article in *Spirituality and Health Magazine*, "Wake Up From Unworthiness," Tara Brach PhD, author of *Radical Acceptance,* wrote, "Many of us spend huge amounts of our lives feeling this way--sometimes it's a very explicit dramatic sense of being damaged goods, and other times, it's a subtle layering of judging ourselves. Whichever it is, it still affects everything. It colors the way we take risks or the way we approach our relationships. We cannot be intimate with another if we are not able to embrace our emotions (Mowe)."

When Ms. Brach teaches her workshops, self-forgiveness and self-compassion are the focus. "We need to have a tender space fully present with our emotions (ibid)." What has happened in our past, such as traumatic events may stay within us and cause difficulties for our health.

Past Traumas

Most of us prefer to bury our emotions deep within us. How do I know this? Because I've done it and most of my patients have also. On the first day of an evaluation, I listen to emotions and past traumas, so my patients know that there may be a direct link from past hurts to present physical pain. Emotional abuse, verbal abuse, physical abuse, and sexual abuse can sometimes remain stuck in our bodies. How our parents treated us then, or still treat us now, how our siblings treated us, how our partners treated us, how we treat ourselves; these all play a role in our pain levels. Letting go of judging ourselves may be the most powerful link to evolving into our higher selves.

"When women open the doors of their own lives and survey the carnage there in those out-of-the-way places, they most often find they have been allowing summary assassinations of their most crucial dreams, goals, and hopes," writes, Clarissa Pinkola Estes, author of *Women Who Run With The Wolves* (Estés, 53).

No wonder it's difficult to evolve; we're held back by our own pain and suffering. We ain't going there. "Not me!" We continue to assassinate our dreams, goals, and hopes. We must find our courage again and let go of our painful emotions, our past.

The rest of this chapter will introduce you to four methods I use to heal emotionally, physically, and spiritually. We must heal our past in order to evolve, my friends.

Four Ways We Can Connect with Emotions and Heal

The four methods which have helped me to heal are John F. Barnes Myofascial Release, journaling, yoga, and Emotional Freedom Techniques. Releasing and honoring our emotional, physical, and spiritual traumas can help heal pain and help us evolve into our next life stanza.

Most of the patients I see have chronic pain. The fascinating common threads are the emotions they've tucked away in their bodies, like carrying heavy baggage. "You are a pain in my neck." You are a pain in my butt." What baggage are we still carrying?

John F. Barnes Myofascial Release (JFB MFR)

In 2006, I took a course in manual therapy that would change my life forever. JFB Myofascial Release is a technique that releases the fascia, or connective tissue, which presents itself as a "tight area," "a painful area," "a feeling of being stuck," "inability to move," "inability to breathe," or just "carrying a heavy, painful load on our shoulders." JFB MFR is a hands-on technique that uses gentle sustained pressure for five minutes or more in these restricted areas. It decreases inflammation, increases range of motion, and allows patients to feel better emotionally and physically.

I've enjoyed many courses with John F. Barnes (Return). My way of life has completely changed. My patients have come along for the ride. John was the first health practitioner or physical therapist I heard say, "We all have the ability to heal ourselves, and we need to connect with that innate power." He was also the first person to introduce me to the healing aspects of physical emotional release. My classes with John are never ending. This cutting-edge manual therapy is so loving and compassionate. After practicing JFB MFR for thirteen years, I am not surprised at how evidence-based research is growing and supporting this work that began 60 years ago.

To understand what fascia is Dr. Carol Davis professor Emerita of The University of Miami Miller School of Medicine discusses in her book, *Integrative Therapies in Rehabilitation; Evidence For Efficacy in Therapy, Prevention, and Wellness,* Dr. Davis writes, "Fascia covers the muscles, bones, nerves, organs, and vessels down to the cellular level. Therefore, malfunction of the system due to trauma, poor posture, or inflammation can bind down the fascia, resulting in abnormal pressure on any or all these body components. It is through that process that this binding down, or restriction may result in many of the poor or temporary results achieved by conventional medical, dental, and therapeutic treatments. Those practicing the JFB MFR approach use the skin and fascia as a handle, or lever, to create new options for enhanced function and movement of every structure of the body. The JFB MFR approach helps to remove the straitjacket of pressure caused by restricted fascia, eliminating symptoms, such as stiffness, pain, and spasms (Davis, 58-59)."

The new idea of using your hands to hold gentle sustained pressure into the fascia for three to five minutes or more was researched by Paul Stanley, PhD and associates from the University of Arizona in Phoenix. This gentle sustained pressure releases healing messenger cells, cytokines and interleukins. In the article, *Get Lasting Results With This Myofascial Technique,* Carol Davis is asked to explain Dr. Stanley's work, " After three minutes there is an increased release of the anti-inflammatory interleukin eight (anti-inflammatory), interleukin three (white blood cell formation) and interleukin oneB (nitric oxide, vasodilation) which all impact tissue recovery and `healing (Probert)."

In his latest edition of *Myofascial Release, Healing Ancient Wounds: The Renegade's Wisdom*, Barnes writes, "You and I as humans are a powerful electromagnetic field of liquid light. Much of this goes back to the incredible insights of Albert Einstein and Nikola Tesla who both stated that everything is energy. When we go through trauma, a vector of force is thrust into our body. This alters the polarity in the traumatized tissue and the energetic flow while altering the vibrational rate. This then changes what should be fluid, the ground substance of fascia, into a more viscous state and eventually a much more solid state capable of crushing pressure. When we apply sustained pressure at the barrier, for a sufficient amount of time, we are allowing the polarity and vibratory rate to return to its norm and in so doing, the system now rehydrates allowing the tissue to glide which ultimately removes the pressure that creates so many of our symptoms and malfunction of our physiology (Barnes, 354)." Bam! This is why I do this work.

When we have pain for a long time, it also breaks us down emotionally. John F. Barnes encourages us to roll up the windows and scream in the car, or into a pillow, hit the bed, jiggle, unwind, or cry. All of it is profoundly healing. Find a John F Barnes trained therapist near you. Mr. Barnes was also the first person to educate me on the healing aspects of writing in a journal.

Journaling

Expressive writing, or journaling, allows for a healthy emotional release. It decreases asthma and rheumatoid arthritis. It also decreases high blood pressure and elevated WBC, white blood cell count. Allowing our emotions, thoughts, and beliefs to leave our physical bodies and be transferred on to paper or the phone or computer, is truly healing.

Here is an excerpt of Dr. Pamela M. Peekes' article, *Reduce Stress by Journaling*

"When life's challenges seem overwhelming, women often find that talking about their stress helps them put it in perspective. However, there's another great way to maintain control of your thoughts and decision making throughout each day: Journaling. I don't mean writing long and detailed stories of your life experiences. Journaling is the simple act of regularly jotting down your life events and feelings on paper-or even at your laptop, desktop, or typewriter. Your journal can help you refine your daily living skills. It gives you the opportunity to reflect on the experiences and events you've recorded. You can use journaling to help you deal with stressors you don't feel comfortable sharing with others. Stress psychologists have shown that journaling enhances immune function and can alter the course of chronic conditions such as rheumatoid arthritis and asthma (Peekes)."

There are many ways to journal, and recommendations are all over the internet for you. They seemed a little too point specific, so I would like to share my own personal way that I journal that hopefully may be a little easier:

• **When to journal?** I make time to write in my journal every morning when I get to work or when I'm at a coffee shop. For some reason the energy and smell of coffee/tea and something baking has always opened my connection with my higher self. I do sometimes like to write in bed before I go to sleep to make sure I'm not worrying about something that I don't need to be worrying about.

• **Where do I keep my journal?** I carry my journal in my purse so I can write anytime.

• **How much time?** In the morning before I see my first patient; it's usually 5-15 minutes. If I'm at a coffee shop it can be 20-45 minutes. In bed it just depends on how late it is and what book I've just read. I don't write in my journal every day, but I notice life runs a little smoother when I do.

• **What should I write?** I always begin with Dear God or Dear Jackie, and then I write what I'm feeling at that moment. Sometimes a dialogue begins with myself and God and sometimes it's just me spilling my guts out. I don't share my journal with anyone, because my writing can get ugly.

• **How do I inspire myself to write?** I read meditation books that inspire me when I take a hot bath in the early morning so my writing will review what sparked my heart or I will focus on a problem or issue that I'm trying to figure out or let go of. I also write down my aspirations and dreams. If I want to manifest something, I usually have to write it on paper first because then it has a better chance of becoming real.

• **Recommendations**: A wonderful journal I have recently started to use and now recommend is "The Five-minute Journal" by Alex Ikonn and UJ Ramdas from Intelligent Change. It has daily quotes and specific questions that keep you on track. Not into paper journaling? Try a journal smartphone app: Penzu Free Diary and Private Journal app.

The third method to release emotions is yoga. In 1849, while living near Walden Pond in Concord, Massachusetts, Henry David Thoreau wrote a letter to his friend H.G.O. Blake about yoga. In it, he said...

"Depend on it that, rude and careless as I am, I would fain practice the yoga faithfully. To some extent, and at rare intervals, even I am a yogi (*Yoga*)." Yes, Thoreau did yoga.

Yoga

The setting is my all-girl high school gym class at St. Agnes in Queens, New York. We wore a special athletic uniform: a tee-shirt and green baggy shorts with elastic on the thighs. By baggy I mean, picture a dark green cotton bag that snaps at your waist, poofs out at the hips, with rubber bands squeezing your legs. Picture a conquistador without tights. I'm guessing the school's goal was to get us to focus less on the flesh and more on the spirit. Our tall gym teacher barked out the words, "Sit on your mats. We are doing yoga today." We all looked at each other wondering, what the heck is yoga? Ms. Gotleib was a tough cookie with a heavy German accent. She yelled again, "Grab the gym mats and sit like me." We walked to the wall and peeled off the grey thick mats from the top of the pile and dragged them over. We sat cross-legged in front of her. She started to take deep breaths and asked us to breathe deeply with her. Then she asked us, a group of teenage girls, to sit quietly and just breathe for the next five minutes. We thought she had lost her mind, but we did what we were told. No one wants to go to the principal's office when the principal is a nun. The first thirty seconds were filled with giggles until she started to say things like "Let your shoulders drop," "Listen to the silence," "Slow your breathing down." My friends were fidgeting, but for me it was the coolest thing ever. I'd never sat quietly in a cross-legged position. Heck, I'd never sat quietly, in complete silence, period. It was so weird, yet it was wonderful at the same time. It felt like the world stopped turning for those few minutes as we breathed deeply.

I remember it was the very first time I was aware of air going in and air going out. Then she asked us to watch her as she did, "Salute to the sun." Sounds funnier if you hear it in a German accent. She stood up, and her arms reached to the sky, then she slowly bent forward with a straight back, arms out like she was flying, and put her hands on the floor, she placed one leg behind her, then the other one, and her butt went up to the sky. It was incredible. How could someone that old do that? She was around forty-five. Ms. Gotleib asked us to try it with her. I looked around and it was like watching everyone do Twister. Hilarious! We asked her what yoga meant and she said, "To keep it simple, yoga means union." We all had a new respect for our gym teacher after that day. I never practiced yoga again until I was living in Manhattan.

"Yoga is the Settling of the Mind into Silence (Chopra)." --The Yoga Sutras

Yoga has always been a big thing in New York City. I practiced it for a while in my late twenties, until I realized it triggered some past dance injuries causing my body to hurt, so I stopped. I didn't realize at the time that yoga brings an awareness to the areas of the body that have fascial restrictions, areas that are tight. Therefore, yoga brings awareness to areas of the body that need your attention and want to be freed.

In Mississippi, my friend Hope Landis invited me to a class she was teaching at River Rock Yoga. The great teacher, Moira Anderson, runs it. I fell in love with yoga again. She made me aware of a yoga that was not just about forcing my body into poses; she taught me how to use blankets, blocks, and bolsters to support my body and make it comfortable. It was a kind and compassionate, uplifting, life-changing feeling. The more I practiced yoga, the calmer and happier I became. Yoga was meditation, but I was moving instead of sitting. For me it was a slow, loving, meditative dance. Some call it meditation in motion.

When I practice yoga every morning, I feel I am connecting to God. It's the coolest, most breathtaking experience. It is even more powerful when I take a class. The energy from the yoga teacher and the students in the class is so loving and kind. I attribute not needing antidepressants to my meditation and yoga practice all these years. I now combine John F Barnes myofascial release self-treatment before, during, and after my yoga practice. I have created a workshop called Myofascialyoga and also created ChakraMFR which both can be used to self treat. If you'd like to see them in video form you can order my online course, "Back and Neck Pain Relief: The Surprising Gut and Brain Connection at: you-can-heal@teachable.com

My beautiful colleague. Grace Vedalia, PT, has coined the term MFR Yoga, and teaches this in her Memphis, Tennessee, practice by the same name.

According to Osteopath Dr. Natalie Nevins, yoga can,

• Lessen chronic pain, such as lower back pain, arthritis, headaches, and carpal tunnel syndrome

• Lower blood pressure

• Reduce insomnia

• Increase flexibility

• Increase muscle strength and tone

• Improve respiration, energy, and vitality

• Maintain a balanced metabolism

• Assist in weight reduction

• Improve cardio and circulatory health

• Improve athletic performance

• Protect from injury

• Relieve chronic stress patterns

• Assist in developing coping skills

• Create a positive outlook on life

• Create mental clarity and calmness (Benefits)

I would like to share a definition of yoga that inspires me by B.K.S Iyengar, author of *Light on Yoga:* "Yoga is the method by which the restless mind is calmed, and the energy directed into constructive channels. As a mighty river, when properly harnessed by dams and canals, creates a vast reservoir of water, prevents famine and provides abundant power for industry: so also the mind, when controlled, provides a reservoir of peace and generates abundant energy for human uplift (Iyengar, 20)."

How do you like that? Pretty awesome, right? I chose Iyengar's quote because his early years were filled with illness until he found yoga. At age fifteen, he had tuberculosis, typhoid fever, and malaria. The doctors said he wouldn't live past the age of twenty. He went to stay with his brother-in-law, who taught him the self-healing techniques of yoga. Guess what? He healed himself through yoga. He then began teaching yoga in other parts of India and later brought hatha yoga to the West.

One of the first physical therapists who talked about yoga in the United States was Judith Hanson Lasseter. She is a founder of The Iyengar Yoga Institute and *Yoga Journal* magazine. She's written nine books, her latest is called *Restore and Balance, Yoga for Deep Relaxation*. In it, she responds to a question about how to encourage oneself to practice yoga. She wrote, "Just set a timer for twenty minutes and get on your mat. I don't care what you do. Maybe you just lie there for twenty minutes. You're going to feel better. Lie there and breathe. People are going to like to be around you more. You'll be more mellow. Just get on the mat. And whatever you do for those twenty minutes, just do it (Yoga)." I love this, and personally invite you to join me.

This reminds me of a personal experience. One day, many years ago during a yoga class, the strangest thing started to happen. I began to cry. I told the teacher afterwards, and she said, "You haven't done true yoga until you've cried during your yoga practice." Wow. I thought I was revealing a hidden flaw, but I was upgrading myself in the yoga world! This was so similar to John F. Barnes' Myofascial Release, that now when I practice yoga, I know it's often called connecting to your mind, body, spirit, and fascia. A good place to help you find a great school or teacher is yoga alliance. Nothing replaces a yoga class where you can ask questions, get feedback, share laughter and energy with others. If you are a healthcare professional check out Ginger Garner PT. She teaches PYT, Professional Yoga Therapy, with tons of evidence-based research that shows that yoga is medicine. I've enjoyed eight of her courses.

Now, let's enter the tapping world. No, not tap dancing. Even though I recommend that too. The fourth way to connect with our emotions and heal is through EFT.

Emotional Freedom Technique (EFT or Meridian Tapping)

One restless night, at 2:00 A.M. to be exact, I started to feel my heart race. I knew it was anxiety. Why was I feeling anxious? Who the heck knows? But my theory is that I was living in the future and sliding into fear, but that's my opinion. I got up to use the restroom, drank some water, took slow deep breaths, and realized it was not going away. I got into bed and started tapping the outside of my palm and other points on my head, face, and upper body for about five minutes, and my heart stopped racing. Then I fell into a beautiful sleep. I knew how to do this because of my wonderful natural physician Betty Sue O'Brian. She did this first with my teenage daughter, and it helped her a lot. So, I started doing it. Later I took a course with Dr. Dawson Church, and I use tapping now with many of my patients.

Emotional Freedom Technique is a healing tool that uses self-tapping on acupuncture meridian end points. In the Eighties, Dr. Roger Callahan had a patient with a water phobia. After exhausting all forms of therapy, he tried tapping, and she was cured. All he asked her to do was think of her fear while tapping under her eye. He termed this, Thought Field Therapy (TFT). Gary Craig took the TFT course with Dr. Callahan and went on to publish the *EFT*

Handbook. Dr. Dawson Church has written the easy-to-read, pocket-size EFT Manual and the EFT for PTSD manual. The US Veterans Administration has approved EFT as a complimentary integrative health practice. This brings me so much joy because it works, and our veterans deserve the best. According to his research, seventy-two genes are enhanced during EFT and 450 neural pathways are also altered. The evidence-based science behind this is so powerful (Church).

Affirmations or words that are used during tapping can be, "Even though I feel_____ (anxiety, fear, self-doubt, lack of confidence, sadness, etc.) I deeply and completely accept myself." This sentence structure is very healing. EFT and similar techniques are often discussed under the umbrella terms "energy medicine/energy psychology." EFT operates on the premise that no matter what part of your life needs improvement, there are underlying negative emotions that need to be addressed. EFT is also recommended for people with past traumas such as sexual abuse ("Home: EFT Universe"). Another way to heal yourself is by choosing the right health care provider to join you on your healing journey. The practitioners you choose can affect your ability to heal more than we care to admit.

Choosing the Right Healthcare Provider

We're living at a great time in medical history. We have more options than ever before when it comes to medical practitioners. Western medical physicians are adding more education for the benefit of themselves and their patients including functional medicine, integrative medicine, natural medicine, herbal/homeopathic, ayurvedic medicine, lifestyle medicine, and iridology. Nutrition and lifestyle changes are now part of the prescription, not just the medications.

Choosing a caring compassionate provider can make the difference between getting better or getting sicker.

Allowing health practitioners to tell us how sick we are and how long we have to live changes our beliefs and diminishes our ability to freely heal. Choosing a healthcare provider is one of the most important decisions we can make. Shop around. We take more time shopping for a car then we do for choosing a doctor. Have a consultation with a minimum of three and see which one resonates with you. How does their website make you feel? Do they shake your hand? Do they look at you? Are they rushing? Which one emits good energy? Which one lifts you up spiritually? Speaking of spiritually, let's walk into the spiritual room.

Come on, you can do it.

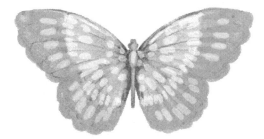

Chapter Five:
'S' The Spiritual Room

Compassion, Kindness, Energy, Power

"The Most Beautiful and Profound Emotion We Can Experience is the Sensation of the Mystical. It is the Power of All True Science" (Favorite Quotations)

--Albert Einstein

This transports me back to a visit I made to the Carmelite Monastery in Mobile, Alabama. As you drive through the wrought iron gates and approach the beautiful brick buildings surrounded by oak and cedar trees, a peace suddenly embraces you. One of my idols has always been Mother Teresa of Calcutta, now a saint, so I feel comfortable in the company of nuns. This visit was not a joyful one or even a contemplative one. It was a specific, what the heck is going on here visit. I wanted to know why my beautiful, loving, caring Aunt Sylvia was dying. She had been diagnosed with pancreatic cancer, and I needed to speak to one of the sisters. As I sat on the other side of a wooden lattice, I could feel the high vibrational energetic field of love and oneness all around me.

As the Carmelite nun, in a brown religious habit walked into the other side of the lattice and sat across from me all I felt from her was what I call, "A Knowing." Here was a human who experiences a field of high vibrational level of oneness, "Holy Spirit" every day. She explained how my aunt was experiencing a mystery. Living with a terminal illness has no rhyme or reason. This is what is called carrying the cross. When we accept this cross, we offer it up to God and this balances the pain and suffering of the world. She went on to explain that cloistered sisters pray and sing every day for peace and healing in the world. This way of life decreases the suffering of the world.

I left the cloistered nun with mixed emotions. I knew that her words carried wisdom, but every cell of my body was resisting. No not resisting, fighting. I was fighting for my aunt's life. I wanted the cross to be lifted from her back. I could care less about balancing the pain and suffering of the world. What about the pain and suffering of her husband, children and our entire family? I wanted the mystery to end with her healing. I wanted God to heal her now!

I went back to NY to visit my aunt, and I repeated the nun's words to her. Her response was also filled with a "knowing," which is the only way I can explain it. She was also grateful. She felt there was a purpose in her life even if it was shrouded in mystery. Her purpose was to accept and carry her cross knowing that she was creating an energetic balance for the world. The closeness and love of her husband, children, and grandchildren was a representation of God's oneness with her during her transition from this human experience.

After Aunt Sylvia's death, I hated and screamed at God for a very long time. I was sick and tired of the mystery. All

I knew was that there was one less angel on this earth, and my uncle, cousins, family, and I were left alone. Then, after a couple of years, my anger with God started to decrease. I accepted the mystery and released my control. It was then that I began to feel her presence. She is now part of the life force, The Holy Spirit, or collective consciousness that flows through the universe. It is what scientists now call, The Field.

Get to Know the Energetic Spirit that you are.

In the book, *The Field: The Quest for the Secret Force of the Universe,* Lynne McTaggart writes about what respected scientists have discovered, "At our most elemental, we are not a chemical reaction, but an energetic charge. Human beings and all living things are a coalescence of energy in a field of energy connected to every other thing in the world. Scientists have provided evidence that all of us connect with each other and the world at the very undercoat of our being. Through scientific experiment they'd demonstrated that there may be such a thing as a life force flowing through the universe - what was called collective consciousness or as theologians have termed it, The Holy Spirit (McTaggart, xviii)."

Wait a minute. Science is now saying that consciousness is a field of energy and it's the Holy Spirit? This means spirituality and science are coming together. As Dr. Lipton reveals, "The fact that scientific principles led me, a non-seeker, to spiritual insight is appropriate because the latest discoveries in physics and cell research are forging new links between the worlds of science and spirit (Lipton, 203)." This consciousness has been mapped out in the next page by Dr. David Hawkins by using numerical energy levels based on truth and falsehood.

"We are Spiritual Beings Having a Human Experience."
--Pierre Teilhard de Chardin

When I first heard this quote by paleontologist and Jesuit priest, Teilhard de Chardin, I felt a profound sensation throughout my body that I can only describe as peace. In this one sentence everything made sense. My body, mind, and spirit are parts of an energy field connected to every other being; it's called consciousness.

"Out beyond ideas of wrongdoing and rightdoing, there is a field. I'll meet you there

-Rumi.

High Vibrational Energy

Dr. David Hawkins, author of <u>Power vs. Force</u>, writes: "In this interconnected universe, every improvement we make in our private world improves the world at large for everyone. We all float on the collective level of consciousness of mankind, so that any increment we add comes back to us. We all add to our common buoyancy by our efforts to benefit life. It is a scientific fact that what is good for you is good for me (David)." In this book Dr. Hawkins created a numerical scale of energy fields of consciousness called the Map of Consciousness. In this scale we can visually see the lower energy levels and their numbers versus the higher energy levels and their numbers.

I will attempt to describe the Map of Consciousness by first giving you a visual of just three of the columns for simplicity. At the bottom of the scale the lowest energy level/emotion is shame/humiliation and measured at 20, above it is guilt/blame 30, apathy/despair 50, grief/regret 75, fear/anxiety 100, desire/craving 125, anger/hate 150, pride/scorn 175. He labels these lower levels as False because understanding is limited, and awareness is low. Once your energy levels rise to 200 which is courage/affirmation you enter higher levels of truth. The consecutive levels above that are neutrality/trust 250, willingness/optimism 310, acceptance/forgiveness 350, reason/understanding 400, love/reverence 500, joy/serenity 540, peace/bliss 600, enlightenment/ineffable 700-1000.

In Dr. Hawkins's own words, "A person in grief which calibrates at the level of 75, will be in a much better condition if he rises to anger, which calibrates at 150. Anger itself, however, is a destructive emotion and is still a low state of consciousness, but as social history shows, Apathy can imprison entire subcultures as well as individuals. If the hopeless can come to wanting something better (Desire at 125) and then use the energy of Anger at 150 to develop Pride at 175, they may then be able to take the step to Courage, which calibrates at 200, and proceed to actually ameliorate their individual or collective conditions. Conversely, the person who has arrived at a habitual state of unconditional Love will experience anything less to be unacceptable (Hawkins 93)."

My main question was how in the world did he calibrate these levels? The answer is twenty years of research and millions of calibrations using kinesiological muscle testing. Kinesiology is the study of body movements. "Clinical Kinesiological muscle testing has found widespread verification over the last twenty-five years. Goodheart's original research on the subject was given wider application by Dr. John Diamond (xxi)." Dr. Hawkins has taken the muscle testing further from a positive and negative response to a truth or false response. The test is simple. You place gentle pressure on the outstretched arm of an individual just above the wrist, while asking her/him a simple true or false question. After repeating the muscle testing millions of times Hawkins was able to calibrate the responses. "Exhaustive investigation has resulted in a calibrated scale of consciousness, in which the log of whole numbers from 1-1,000 calibrates the degree of power of all possible levels of human awareness (xii)."

While reading his book it dawned on me that the muscle testing is compressing on the web of connective tissue, fascia, which touches each cell membrane in our body. The cell membrane has microtubules which scientists believe to be connected to consciousness. "Similar to Einstein, anesthesiologist Dr. Stuart Hammeroff's intuition showed him that there were tiny structures in our cells called microtubules, which could explain consciousness. He was joined by Sir Roger Penrose, one of the most esteemed figures in mathematical physics. Through years of work they developed a theory called 'Orchestrated Objective Reduction,' which suggests that structures called microtubules could transport materials and chemicals inside cells and underlies our conscious thinking. They believe quantum physics might be vital to our cognition and even memory (Barnes 12)."

This brings me back to our connective tissue, fascia, that is being tested by gentle pressure in the kinesiological tests. If our consciousness is in our microtubules of the fascia, which is part of the cell membrane, then that's how we get true or false answers during the testing.

John F Barnes PT, first visualized this 50 years ago as he explains, "My intuition (channel 3) guided me both through visual images and instinctive 'felt sense' revealing to me how the fascial system is not an insulator, but a semiconductor and how every fascial fiber down to the tiniest of levels is actually a microtubule with a hollow core. Within the hollow core is fluid, and within the fluid flows photons which are the primary communication of our body at the cellular level (12)."

We now go back to epigenetics where genes do not control life, but rather our thoughts or consciousness, what we believe, located in the cell membrane, controls life.

In his book, *The Biology of Belief,* Dr. Bruce Lipton expresses his moment of insight when he connected his lifelong studies of the cell membrane to the "Spirit." "I ran wild-eyed into the medical library because of a flash of life-changing insight concerning the nature of the cell membrane that was downloaded into my awareness in the wee hours of the morning. In assessing the beauty and elegance of the membrane's mechanics, I was drawn to the conclusion that we are immortal, spiritual beings who exist separately from our bodies. I had heard an undeniable inner voice informing me that I was leading a life based not only on the false premise that genes control biology but also on the false premise that we end when our bodies die. I had spent years studying molecular control mechanisms within the physical body and at that astounding moment came to realize that the protein 'switches' that control life are primarily turned on and off by signals from the environment, the Universe.

You may be surprised that it was science that led me to that moment of spiritual insight. These realms were split apart in the days of Descartes centuries ago. However, I truly believe that only when Spirit and Science are reunited will we be afforded the means to create a better world (Lipton, 202)." This is one reason why I wrote this book. I've noticed when I allow myself to connect with this field that I also call Holy Spirit, my body responds physiologically, pain decreases, and I feel better and more connected. This is the high vibrational frequency of love and the levels above, when I venture to reach even higher.

Love

"We do not exist for ourselves alone, and it is only when we are fully convinced of this fact that we begin to love ourselves properly and thus also love others." Thomas Merton (Thomas)

On a snowy Christmas Eve, at my mother's NYC apartment, my boyfriend of four years Scott, shocked me with an engagement ring in front of my entire family. I thought there were no more gifts because he had already given me what I asked for, a self-install jacuzzi. Do you remember those? You unfolded this three-tiered plastic compartmental thingamajig, placed it on the bottom of the tub and pushed down so that the six suction cups would adhere. Then connected a hose to a motor and when your bathtub was full you turned it on and voila, instant jacuzzi. I was so excited and made such a big deal about it that my mean aunt Connie who wore diamonds and gold to just pick up the mail made the comment, "Wow, what a big deal you're making over this jacuzzi. I can't imagine how you're going to respond when you get a ring." I quickly glanced at her and said, "Scott knows I don't want a ring."

Meanwhile, there was one more gift, and it was inside the Christmas tree. He grabbed it and came close to me so quickly I didn't have time to see what he was doing. He stood to the left of me and stretched out his arms as he opened the little black velvet box. All eyes were on me. No one breathed in the small living room because I wasn't breathing! My aunt for the first time said nada. Finally, I looked into his eyes and said, "What is this?" Scott said, "Well, what do you think it is?" No, he didn't get down on his knee. I said, "I don't think I can accept this." Scott said, "Okay, I'll take it back," he smiled and sat down in my grandmother's rocking chair. I ran to my bedroom so my whole family could breathe again. Scott came after me and saw how frightened I was. I kept asking him why he gave me a ring, and he said since we were together for a long time it was a sign to my family that he loved me. He also said if I didn't want it to be an engagement ring it could be a friendship ring. I think he was freaking out that I was so terrified, as fear is not something he was used to seeing in me.

I called my Mom and Mawelita into my room and explained the ring was a sign of Scott's love for me and nothing else. My mother and grandmother just smiled and said, "How nice." As the wise women they were, they knew we would be married, but they didn't want to freak me out even more. Dance was always my priority, and luckily, I had found someone who honored that. I was not ready for my priorities to be about a man.

Interestingly though, I started to look at my ring all the time. I even began to wear white clothes. It was as if the ring had some magical powers. I was noticing some subtle changes within me. I also started to feel our relationship changing. I was more, "in Love." I didn't know it then, but my vibrational frequency level of consciousness was higher. I was happier and smiled more. It felt at times like I was glowing. Then, that word kept creeping up in my head, marriage. Marriage? I don't believe in marriage. Who invented this word? Where does it come from? Did a man invent it? Who in their right mind would invent such a ridiculous thing? A woman must enter into a contract to be with only one man for the rest of her life. Are you kidding me? So why was I thinking about it so much? What was happening to me? Was I becoming weak? Then a little voice in my head said, "What are you afraid of?" I responded, "Being with the same person until I die, doing someone else's laundry, compromising on everything for the rest of my life. Impossible."

I only knew of two people who remained married: my grandmother, whose husband died before I was born, so they were only married for thirty-five years--divorce was not an option for women in South America before the 1960's--and my uncle, who married an angel, Sylvia. Everyone else in my family had been divorced at least once. It was then I realized I was changing. A little piece of my new wing was pushing through the top of the cocoon. I was evolving. I was falling in love. No wait, not falling, but becoming love. I didn't know that when you enter higher vibrational frequencies you "Be-Come" those frequencies. You allow yourself to "Be" in the moment of that frequency and then it "Comes" and floods every cell of your body. This changes you physiologically.

With some sleepless nights, and some crying, I had the courage to remove my fear of marriage. I gave myself permission to marry Scott, my fiancé, but I moved into an apartment in Manhattan for a year first, because I wanted to know what it was like to be on my own. Latina women usually go from mama's house to the husband's house.

After leaving dance, accepting the ring on my finger was not a friendship ring, and moving into Manhattan on the Upper Westside; I got my first full time job. I was fortunate to get a position as a concierge at the New York Marriott

Marquis Hotel at Times Square. What's a concierge? That's exactly what I said. The definition is "the keeper of the keys and someone who answers your questions." In New York City, however, it means, "Anything you need I will get it for you or make it magically appear." I had previous experience at the Midway hotel in Queens, thanks to Joe Martelli. I was fluent in Spanish and communicated in French, and of course, my college degree was a big help. I loved being a concierge of my hometown. As I was settling into my position of non-dancing concierge woman, I was also settling into the interesting fiancée life.

After about three months of this new life, Scott and I started arguing. We weren't used to seeing each other all the time. I was no longer leaving for my 10:00 A.M. ballet class or voice lesson or jazz class or audition. I didn't leave to go perform for a couple of months. We were with each other a lot. Amazingly, we got through the stressful transition of the engagement period.

We were happily married a year later, in 1989, when I was twenty-seven. That first year we ate out often, and I gained a lot of weight. I was enjoying the world of newlyweds, but was not connected to myself and just went through the motions of living without any regard for my body. The weight gain made me sad. I was then at the other end of the pendulum. I went from a skinny, unhealthy dancer to a chubby, unhealthy housewife. Something in me stirred, and I felt I wanted to be a physical therapist again, but then I remembered, "I wasn't smart enough and wasn't good enough." Since one needs two jobs to afford Manhattan, I took a course and became a personal trainer in Long Beach, Long Island, with the help of ECA, East Coast Alliance. Thank you, Carol and Scott Lapidus. I learned how to exercise and eat healthy for the first time. I lost the weight I had gained, and even became an aerobics instructor. Anyone remember your first step class in the late Eighties to the early Nineties? Ask your knees, they remember everything.

I convinced myself that a personal trainer was the nearest I would ever get to becoming a physical therapist because I wasn't smart enough or good enough. A year later, I became the only female trainer allowed on "the floor" at World Gym at Lincoln Center. I was happy with my life. I was not a physical therapist, but I was close enough. At work, my favorite part was calling my clients' physical therapists and conferring with them on the clients' exercise therapy. I remember one physical therapist's voice was strong, smart, all-knowing, and kind. Nothing like mine. However, I do remember understanding everything he said, and I even made recommendations which he approved. A little voice, God, would say, "See, you are pretty smart." My quick reply was, "No, I am not. I could never be like them!" During this time my Mawelita was in a lot of pain, so one night my mom called and said to meet her in the ER, Mawelita was not well.

Dr. Hawkins tells us that in hopeless untreatable cases, recovery has been due to a major shift in consciousness, "In spontaneous recovery there is frequently a marked increase in the capacity to love and the awareness of the importance of love as a healing factor and modality (Hawkins, 240)."

The setting is the ER room at Queens Elmhurst hospital. Grandma (Mawelita) is 92 years young with severe abdominal pain. I'm crying and holding my little Mawelita's thin, wrinkled hands. ER rooms are overcrowded and scary in NYC. The EMT's transferred her from the ambulance stretcher to another stretcher in the cold hallway. They gave the nurse all her vitals and left quickly. After several x rays and nurses trying to kick me out, they let me stay because I was the only translator available. A doctor appears and says, "Your grandmother needs her gallbladder removed as soon as possible, but she may die during surgery." God bless doctors because they sure don't know how to break it to you gently. Now, if you know me at all you know my grandma is everything to me. My mom and I approved the surgery for the next morning. The next day, two new doctors, one of Indian descent and the other Jewish, came into her Pre-Op room and spoke to us. Standing at the foot of her bed they began to speak, "This surgery is going to be very difficult for her body because of her age. We don't know how she'll react during and after the surgery, but she is a very healthy woman otherwise and she can very easily do well, or she may not survive the surgery." After I translated their words to her she responded by saying, "I am in God's hands and God will guide your hands."

Oh my Gosh. Now, I had to tell them her exact words. I wanted to add, "No pressure, huh?" After I translated her exact words, they did something remarkable. They bowed their heads in prayer, and one of them touched her foot! They didn't say they were praying they just bowed their heads and closed their eyes. It was about six seconds of what I felt was divine love; it was a "Holy" moment. You could feel the energy in that room change instantly. My mom and I were in shock. The energy shifted from a scientific, medical moment to a holy, divine, love-filled moment. We were all letting go and letting God. We were accepting whatever the outcome would be.

I hugged and kissed Mawelita and entered the mystery of the outcome, before she was wheeled away into the operating room. We entered the waiting area and watched TV for hours with other families. Finally, both doctors came back with a relieved look on their faces and said, "Your grandmother did very well. We'll keep an eye on her for a couple of days and then she can go home." I grabbed each one in my arms and hugged them so tightly and thanked them profusely. To this day I truly believe the doctors level of consciousness rose after they heard my grandmother's words. I believe that when we give ourselves permission to enter into higher levels of vibrational frequencies of trust, love, and oneness we enter the divine infinite possibilities of healing.

Letting go of fear is also a way to create a major shift in consciousness or community of consciousness.

A Community of Consciousness

In Dr. Lipton's article, *Why and How to Let Go of Fear,* he writes,

"Each of us is living in a field of energy, and each of us contributes to that energy through our consciousness. Each human is like a tuning fork whose brain is vibrating at a specific frequency. Therefore, a whole community can vibrate in harmony, as in a community sharing yoga. By definition, the collective community manifests an energy field that is powerful and palpable enough to support the individuals sharing that field. When you experience this energy, it has reassuring and calming effects that will make you want to stay in this field. And increasing the size of the field is clearly the evolutionary path toward a sustainable new humanity (Lipton)."

"Compassion and kindness, it turned out, was good for your health."

James R. Doty

Acts of Altruism

In 1851, the term Altruism was coined by French philosopher Auguste Comte, *altruisme* meaning moral acts intended to promote the happiness of others or self-sacrifice for the benefit of others. How is altruism beneficial for your health? How is it not beneficial?

James R. Doty, M.D., FACS, FICS, is a Clinical Professor of neurosurgery at Stanford University, and founder and director of the Center for Compassion and Altruism Research and Education. He has written a book called, *Into the Magic Shop: A Neurosurgeon's Quest to Discover the Mysteries of the Brain and The Secrets of The Heart.* He states in a TEDxSacramento Talk, "We are hardwired to care, recognize suffering in others, and alleviate that suffering (Doty)." He also goes on to say that when we go into the fight/flight/freeze response of our sympathetic nervous system, we feel stress, anxiety, depression, but when we are compassionate, we reverse that and our heart rate and blood pressure decrease, our immune system increases, stress hormone levels return to baseline and the frontal areas of the brain work better. This also occurs when we sit for fifteen minutes, slowly breathing in and out, and focus on compassion. Now that is pretty awesome!.

As a sixth-grade girl in Catholic school, I was given an assignment by my teacher. She was a wonderful, tiny, dressed in full habit, Carmelite Nun. Her words were, "Bring back canned goods for the hungry tomorrow." My interpretation was, "Bring back all the canned goods you have for the hungry." Once she uttered these words, an exhilaration ran through me as if I had been given the most important mission of my life. I remember an electrifying shock of joy running through my body. Of course, we all must feed the hungry.

There should never be anyone hungry! Since my mother left very early for work and my grandmother never questioned the orders of a nun, I scooted the step-up ladder and climbed up to the cupboard. I put every canned good I could fit into a large paper bag and somehow carried it four New York City blocks to St. Joan of Arc Elementary School. To this day, I do not remember my arms hurting or any feeling of inconvenience. All I felt was complete happiness that the hungry were going to eat. I visualized hundreds of people opening the cans and eating. It was awesome, and it changed me forever. I was hooked on compassion and giving. The feeling is still in every cell of my body.

I do remember however, that feeling of discomfort when my classmates only brought two or three cans of food as I plopped my almost ripping bag onto her desk. That feeling disappeared when the nun smiled and thanked all of us equally. It was a lesson for all that each one of us made a difference. My mom had another opinion when she opened the cupboards that evening.

One of the ways I truly believe we can enhance our health is through giving of our time to make the world a better place. A great way to give our time is by giving it first to ourselves. Time spent sitting quietly and meditating has profound effects on stress.

Meditation and Stress

A simple kindness to ourselves and an important stress reliever that I recommend to my physical therapy patients is meditation. Why meditation? Because it decreases pain and relieves stress. In *You Are Not Your Pain* by V. Burch and D. Penman, the authors write, "Mindfulness meditation can decrease chronic pain by fifty-seven percent. Accomplished meditators can reduce it by ninety percent (Burch,). "

Meditation changes your body biochemically and places you smack into your "heal good and feel good" place. For me personally, peace comes over me after I meditate. I feel a weight has been lifted. I feel physically and spiritually better, closer to God, the universe, and the source. For me, prayer is speaking to God and meditation is sitting in silence and listening. It's a great stress reliever. Why do we want to decrease stress and specifically chronic stress?

Chronic stress negatively affects your hormones, intestines, immune system, all your organs, and your ability to detox.

Chronic stress is our response to prolonged emotional pressure. We begin to feel we have little or no control over what's occurring in our lives. Inability to pay bills, a difficult relationship, work issues, and mourning a death are some examples.

"We are just beginning to understand the ways that stress influences a wide range of diseases of aging including heart disease, metabolic syndrome, type two diabetes, and certain types of disability, even early death," writes Sheldon Cohen. A professor of psychology at Carnegie Mellon University in Pittsburgh, he has been at the forefront of stress research for thirty years (Agnvall).

Other conditions that may be caused by chronic stress are the common cold, weight gain, slower healing, sleep dysfunction, depression, ulcers and other stomach problems. Chronic stress can also allow cancer to grow. According to Anil K. Sood, M.D., professor of Gynecologic Oncology and Reproductive Medicine at M.D. Anderson, "Stress hormones can inhibit a process called anoikis, which kills diseased cells and prevents them from spreading. Chronic stress also increases the production of certain growth factors that increase your blood supply. This can speed the development of cancerous tumors (Head)."

According to neuroendocrinologist Dr. Robert Sapolsky, Professor of Biological Sciences, Neurology and Neurological Sciences at Stanford University, there is evidence that chronic stress shrinks neurons in the hippocampus, a part of the brain involved in learning capacity, memory, and positive mood. The self-healing hippocampus has the ability to regenerate, if stress is discontinued (Sapolsky).

How does Meditation Decrease Stress?

Practicing meditation reduces the activity in the sympathetic nervous system, fight or flight, and increases activity in the parasympathetic nervous system, rest and digest. Meditation affects the relationship between these parts of the brain: the amygdala, responsible for stress responses, and the prefrontal cortex, which can aid in relaxation. The amygdala responds automatically to fear and the front of the brain, when we meditate, calms the amygdala. A good example: your dog hears a noise and starts to bark, (in this case the amygdala), and you, (the front of the brain), get up, to let it know everything is ok. People who meditate bark less.

The Brain Actually Grows during Meditation

In January of 2011, Dr. Sara Lazar, PhD Neuroscience of Yoga and Meditation published the results of a study of meditation on the brain. She and the Harvard Medical School team found that "The brain regions associated with attention and sensory processing were thicker in meditators than in the controls. These findings provide the first evidence that alterations in brain structure are associated with meditation practice. The frontal lobes are interconnected with the limbic system of the brain, the ancient center responsible for both emotions and survival instincts. As the frontal lobes receive messages, they interpret them and signal the limbic system to produce the appropriate emotional responses (The Alternative)."

Dr. Richard Davidson asked the Dalai Lama to allow him to do research with MRI on the brains of the Buddhist monks while they were meditating. The findings were pretty cool:

- Meditation can beneficially change the inner workings and circuitry of the brain, better known as neuroplasticity.
- The happier parts of the brain (prefrontal cortex) were far more active.
- Their brains tend to "re-organize," which means they feel a sense of "oneness" with the world around them.
- The brain wave patterns of the Buddhist monks were far more powerful.
- Their brains had enhanced focus, memory, learning, consciousness, and "neural coordination".
- The monks had no anxiety, depression, addiction, or anything of the sort.

In short, the Buddhist monks' brains were physically and functionally superior to those without meditation experience (7 Fascinating).

Therefore, if you want a free way to have a better memory and a more satisfying, happier, fulfilling, evolving life; sitting quietly and breathing slowly is waiting for you.

How to Begin Meditating

Sit comfortably in a chair or on a cushion on the floor, and count your breaths for one, two, or three minutes. This is how I began to meditate. Setting an intention or a mantra keeps the mind focused. Examples are "I am calm," "I am at peace," "I am connecting with joy," "I love and accept myself." Think or say your mantra as you inhale for four counts and exhale for four counts. This allows your mind to focus on breathing instead of thinking. If thoughts pop up, then just finish the thought and let it float away like a cloud and return to counting the breaths and stating your intention. It's normal for the brain to wander off and think while meditating, so don't worry that you're not doing it correctly.

Simply trying to meditate has tremendous benefits. Allow the thoughts to come. Some of my best ideas have come during meditation. Counting each breath is really helpful. Maybe just start with a goal of ten slow breaths, then work your way up. A great meditation phone app is Headspace. A form of meditation that I use a lot is the Relaxation Response.

Morning and Night, Try the Relaxation Response

Although meditation has been practiced for thousands of years, the meditative technique called the "relaxation response" was pioneered in the U.S. by Harvard cardiologist Dr. Herbert Benson in the Seventies. The technique has gained acceptance by physicians and therapists worldwide as a means of relieving symptoms of conditions ranging from cancer to AIDS (Meditation).

According to Dr. Benson, "The relaxation response is a physical state of deep rest that changes the physical and emotional responses to stress, e.g., decreases in heart rate, blood pressure, rate of breathing, and muscle tension." He adds that, "Deep breathing increases the supply of oxygen to your brain and stimulates the parasympathetic nervous system, which promotes a state of calmness. Breathing techniques help you feel connected to your body. It brings your awareness away from the worries in your head and quiets your mind."

Dr. Benson's stress antidote has practitioners sit quietly for twenty minutes, filling their minds with a positive phrase or belief, and focusing on relaxing their muscles from the feet all the way up to the head. Studies have shown that the Relaxation Response was able to help with many different ailments, from high blood pressure to infertility to rheumatoid arthritis and pain (Dr. Herbert).

Yoga teacher, Frank Jude Bocco explains the difference between relaxation and meditation: "True relaxation is something that is practiced and cultivated; it is defined by the stimulation of the relaxation response. Some forms of conscious relaxation may become meditation, and many meditators find that their practice benefits from using a relaxation technique to access an inner stillness helpful for meditating. Ultimately, it all comes down to the intention and purpose of the technique (Boccio)."

The tides are turning for some of us health care practitioners. We are choosing to work together with primary care physicians and learn more about lifestyle changes and empowering our patients to heal themselves. This means asking the question, "Do I still need that medication"?

Medication or Meditation: Is the Spiritual Room Also Connecting with and Trusting in Your Own Ability to Heal?

After I received my physical therapist license, I started working with a wonderful therapist, Keith Ganey, who had been mentoring me since before I went to PT school. After two weeks at the new job, Hurricane Katrina hit the Gulf Coast on August 29, 2005. The entrance to his PT practice was not passable, so he graciously continued to pay me even though I wasn't working. Who does that? He did.

I proceeded to find work at a skilled nursing facility, SNF, to remove his burden. The facility had triple occupancy as it housed many of the displaced elderly from nursing homes that were destroyed. However, many of their staff had lost their homes and cars as well, and were not able to come to work. For a while, those of us fortunate to have homes and cars were able to come to work and do much more than we ever thought we would as medical professionals.

I had received excellent training from my PT school and at Ocean Springs Hospital in wound therapy from a clinical I did, so I continued on and fell in love with my geriatric patients and their physical and bed sore needs.

Part of the good training I received in the PT master's program was to read past medical history, PMH, and the medication section before I went in for an evaluation. I was shocked to see fifteen to twenty-five medications listed on patients' charts. Why were these elderly people on so many medications? Weren't they having side effects? What was occurring in their livers, kidneys, and brains? I flashed back to the first day in my Anatomy and Physiology class at the University of South Alabama. Dr. Chen walked in, and after he introduced himself, he said these words, "Never forget that every drug you give your patients will have a side effect." He was speaking to all the soon-to-be medical students and nurses in my class, but as a soon-to-be PT, I heard him loud and clear.

I vowed at that moment to start asking questions in care plan meetings with the other medical practitioners, such as nurses, occupational therapists, speech pathologists, CNA's, social workers, and doctors. We all started noticing that once we worked together and listened to the patient, some of the medications were no longer needed.

What made the difference was we became a family. We were touching our patients more and laughing with them more. There was one nurse everyone loved, Nurse Bonnie. She told the patients jokes and made us all laugh. I noticed our patients walking better and looking forward to coming to rehab. CNAs started saying the patients were easier to transfer from bed to wheelchair. It was a time that changed me forever. It taught me that reading a chart thoroughly, touching, hugging, laughing, and loving were all part of a patient's healing. It was part of all our healing.

This was also when I learned that music allowed the patients with dementia and Parkinson's to get up and move easier, and dance! I finally knew why my previous life as a dancer was to help with my patients. It even helped in the ICU or acute care when patients would say, "I don't want to walk" and I would say, "Okay, would you like to dance instead?" This made them smile and everything would change. I would begin to hum a tune and off we'd go. Sit to stand, then stand to dance. Every stanza we leave behind is never wasted. It is there for us to stand on and support us. It is our foundation to share with others.

In Joe Dispenza's book, *You Are the Placebo,* he explains meditation as a substitute for medication, "Instead of taking a pill to change your state of being, you'll be going inward to do it. In time, your meditation will become like your belief in taking medication (Dispenza, 267). This is very dear to my heart because many of my female patients and many women in general are on opioids, antidepressants, and anti-anxiety drugs. One of my main goals as a physical therapist is to offer my patients choices and to bring them to a new level of awareness, so they can share more with their doctors. The awareness of our own ability to heal ourselves and decrease our dependence on medications is truly empowering and can be shared with all of our medical practitioners.

Connecting with the Spiritual 'Body'

In her CNN article, *Are Drugs Stifling Women?* Julie Holland tells us

"Welcome to the increasingly altered states of America. Americans are about five percent of the world's population, yet we take half its pills, and eighty percent of its painkillers. This over-medication has led to record numbers of opiate overdoses and also to a growing number of women taking antidepressants--one out of four and counting, according to a report issued by the pharmacy benefit manager, Medco, certain antidepressants called SSRIs, or selective serotonin reuptake inhibitors, create artificially stable and elevated levels of serotonin, a brain chemical that helps regulate mood, which can dampen empathy and emotional reactivity, while higher doses can engender apathy.

Women are naturally moody. Our moods change, and this emotional fluidity helps us to be adaptable and resilient. We are dynamic and responsive to our environment. There is a biological advantage to this sensitivity; we need to know what our nonverbal babies need, what our mates are thinking and to sense danger in our surroundings. Moodiness -- being sensitive, caring deeply and occasionally being acutely dissatisfied -- is actually a natural source of power. I ensure not only our survival, but that of our o Women's emotionality is a sign of health, not disease, and it is our single biggest psychological asset (Holland)."

A courageous psychiatrist leading the way to changing our addiction to medications is a practicing psychiatrist, Dr. Kelly Brogan. She holds a degree in cognitive neuroscience from MIT, an MD from Weill Cornell Medical College, and clinical training from NYU School of Medicine. In her book, *A Mind of Your Own,* she focuses on drug-free methods that are entirely evidence based. She is passionate about the effectiveness of a holistic and drug-free medicine approach to heal our minds, moods, and memory. Dr. Brogan's approach to depression is encouraging everyone to look, not just in the brain, but for the root cause.

Depression

At one time, someone very dear to me was suffering from depression. Little did I know that the gut problems, bloating, abdominal pain, and not being able to have a bowel movement were contributing to the mood disorder. The doctor's solution was to take Prozac. The solution actually ended up being to heal this person's gut.

I would like to share a new way of looking at depression. Let's look at it from the gut and brain perspective. Since almost every neurotransmitter, the chemical messengers that tell us what mood we're in, is made in our intestines why not look at the gut and brain connection?

According to Dr. Brogan, "Depression is a grossly misdiagnosed and mistreated condition today. Especially amongst women--one in seven of whom is being medicated. One in four women in their forties and fifties use psychiatric drugs. We owe most of our mental illnesses--including their kissing cousins such as chronic worry, fogginess, and crankiness to lifestyle factors and undiagnosed psychological conditions that develop in places far from the brain such as the gut and thyroid," wrote Dr. Brogan (Brogan, 2).

It turns out that it may not be all in your head, but rather in the interconnectedness among the gut, immune and endocrine systems. (Brogan, 23). Our twenty-five feet of intestines contain ninety percent of our immune system, and almost every known neurotransmitter. The neuroendocrine system, the endocrine cells and Enteric nervous system in the intestinal wall, and the endocrine system, which includes glands located from our head to our pelvis, has eight parts. Three glands are in our brain: hypothalamus, pituitary, and pineal glands.

The five other parts are located down the body. In the neck are the thyroid and parathyroid, above the heart nestled between the lungs is the thymus, while the adrenals sit above the kidneys, like little French berets, in the mid-back. The pancreas is below the liver between the kidneys, and the ovaries or testes live in the pelvic region.

Our intestines, gut mucosa, contain endocrine cells, the first line of defense against pathogens. The bacteria in our intestinal walls produce most of the common neurotransmitters found in the brain (Dinan). Bam, the gut and brain connection.

Psychoneuroimmunology and HPA

What do you get when you put together psychological processes, the nervous system and immune systems? PNI, psychoneuroimmunology. Why is this important for your health? Your microbiome that lives in your gut where most of your immune system lives, makes the neurotransmitters that determine your mood. Your little-known microbiome is a hidden community that can make you happy or sad. Think of driving down a road you've never taken and suddenly there's a subdivision that you haven't noticed before hidden away with trillions of people working and living there. That's your microbiome living in the winding roads of your 25 feet of intestines! What's remarkable is when you drive through this subdivision there's an outlet that leads to the mall, for our purposes the brain. These people are bringing stuff that the mall needs twenty-four hours a day. PNI has uncovered something very important called the HPA axis.

HPA (Hypothalamus, pituitary, adrenal) axis is the Hypothalamus which connects the endocrine system to the nervous system that tells the Pituitary to start or stop making hormones and then tells the Adrenal glands to make more or less adrenalin, the fight or flight hormone. Your adrenal glands look like little French hats that sit on top of your kidneys. Fight or flight is where we don't want to hang out for too long. When we hang out there for too long it affects our bowels. When you're not pooping, or the reverse diarrhea, also called IBS, irritable bowel syndrome, it affects your serotonin levels, which affect your sense of well-being and happiness (Alschuler).

Now, to put everything together, if your gut is not working well then it affects your mental health. How can you heal your gut? I'm not a doctor, naturopath, or nutritionist, but when I do the research it appears that staying away from processed foods, eating more plant based foods, avoiding sugar, and drinking filtered water that takes out contaminants such as fluoride and other chemicals, your gut and brain axis heals. Also, if you are not pooping every day the size of a banana it will affect the level of anxiety and may cause depression. After all of this crazy info you may need a nap right now.

What Happens if You Nap for More than Twenty Minutes?

In Jennifer Soong's article, "The Secret and Surprising Power of Naps," she writes "Research shows longer naps help boost memory and enhance creativity. Napping for thirty-sixty minutes is good for decision making skills, such as memorizing vocabulary or recalling directions. Sixty to ninety minutes of napping plays a key role in making new connections in the brain and solving creative problems (Soong)."

Naps or Coffee?

According to Sara C. Mednick PhD, author of *Take A Nap! Change Your Life,* caffeine actually decreases memory performance, whereas power naps have short-term and long-term benefits.

Short-term benefits:

• Sharpens cognitive skills

• Elevates energy levels

• Improves mathematical and logical reasoning

• Increases reaction time

• Improves motor skills

 Long-term benefits:

• Reduces stress

• Decreases the risk of heart disease

• Helps in weight management (Mednick, 23)

Pretty powerful stuff. I believe we need to adopt a siesta time in the USA. The need to simply rest or take an actual nap can also be the fluctuations of our hormones.

Premenstrual Truth/Menopause

With every patient that I see, I refuse to look at their age on the evaluation form. I do this specifically because their number is not a description of who they are, it's society's description.

When I was around 48, I started to feel tired and thought it was because we had three active teenagers. My breasts were tender, my sleep was off, and I was tired all the time. A couple of years later I started to bleed heavily for two weeks during my menstrual cycle and could barely get out of bed. A light bulb went on in my head, and I said, "Oh, this must be menopause." I started to eat better, decrease my wine and sugar intake, but the bleeding continued. I ended up getting blood work done, and my doctor said my iron levels were three! Normal is 8.9-26mcmol/L. Off I went to my gynecologist to get an internal and external ultrasound.

Results were a cyst on each ovary and a uterine fibroid. The left ovary cyst was measured at 2.5 cm and the right ovary was measured at 3.5 cm with the uterine fibroid measuring at 6.0 cm. He recommended a hysterectomy. I asked him if he thought I could get cancer, and he said, "No, your cysts do not have cancer and fibroids are not cancerous." I told him I would check with my natural physician because I was not ready to lose my uterus and ovaries. He had heard of Betty Sue O'Brian, so he agreed. Betty Sue did a complete evaluation that included iridology and sclerology. Iridology is the analysis of the colored part of your eye, the iris, where you can see the inherent strengths and weaknesses of the body. Sclerology is the analysis of the red lines in the white of the eye and shows us the current state of congestion and irritation (Academy).

Betty Sue referred me to a master herbalist, Darrel Martin, and he put me on three herbs that were specific for me. I am also an internal pelvic physical therapist, so I focused on decreasing the size of my cysts and fibroid with myofascial release. In two weeks, my bleeding stopped, and in three months I went back to my gynecologist. The internal ultrasound showed a third decrease in size in my cysts and fibroid. My gynecologist was surprised, and I returned three months later again for an internal ultrasound and cysts and fibroids were so small that he said I didn't have to return until the following year.

I hope this empowers you to seek answers from a natural physician that is well respected in your area. I thankfully have all of my female body parts because I chose to connect my health care providers to each other. The first person to teach me to look elsewhere for answers was gynecologist/obstetrician, Dr. Christian Northrup.

Dr. Christiane Northrup has been a great influence in my life. *The Wisdom of Menopause* was the first book of hers I read. The way she writes allows women to understand their bodies and the reasoning behind our hormone changes and the natural healthy rhythm of our lives. Hearing her describe premenstrual syndrome, PMS, as premenstrual truth, PMT, as well as menopause has been quite an eye opener (Brogan). I have been sharing this truth with everyone. Dr. Northrup's talks about an encoded wisdom during menopause, "It's a passage into the wisdom years, a capacity to open to constant intuitive knowing, reseeding the community (Northrup, *Women's Bodies*, 102)."

Science is Great, but How can I Apply it?

Acknowledge that you are an energetic being connected to all other beings in the world.

Stay in the high vibrational frequency levels of truth: courage, neutrality, willingness, acceptance, reason, love, joy, peace, and enlightenment. Are your thoughts at this moment part of those high frequencies? If not, then it's time to let go of the lower frequencies of fear, anger, judgment, so your thoughts can rise into love and oneness. Feel compassion and be altruistic. Acknowledge your stress levels and decrease them. Take out your calendar and look at the rest of this week. Write or type in:

- Three to ten minutes of meditation every day, which can be done sitting up in bed.
- Yoga class at a beautiful studio with a trained teacher, or at home through an app on your phone or computer, two times a week.
- Walk for twenty or thirty minutes three to four times a week after work or at lunch time.
- Do anything outdoors and have fun.
- Tip: a yoga class knocks out both AST (Active Self Time) and the Relaxation Response.
- Use smartphones to meditate, e.g., Headspace.
- Listen to mindfulness podcasts, such as those found at Hay House, or Connect to Love.
- Honor your evolution through each premenstrual truth, perimenopausal time, or in the freedom of menopause.

Let's end Chapter Five with a poem Charlie Chaplin wrote on his seventieth birthday.

AS I BEGAN TO LOVE MYSELF

As I began to love myself, I found that anguish and emotional suffering are only warning signs that I was living against my own truth. Today, I know, this is "AUTHENTICITY."

As I began to love myself I understood how much it can offend somebody if I try to force my desires on this person, even though I knew the time was not right and the person was not ready for it, and even though this person was me. Today I call it "RESPECT."

As I began to love myself, I stopped craving for a different life, and I could see that everything that surrounded me was inviting me to grow. Today I call it "MATURITY."

As I began to love myself, I understood that at any circumstance, I am in the right place at the right time, and everything happens at the exact right moment. So, I could be calm. Today I call it "SELF-CONFIDENCE."

As I began to love myself, I quit stealing my own time, and I stopped designing huge projects for the future. Today, I only do what brings me joy and happiness, things I love to do and that make my heart cheer, and I do them in my own way and in my own rhythm. Today I call it "SIMPLICITY."

As I began to love myself, I freed myself of anything that is not good for my health – food, people, things, situations, and everything that drew me down and away from myself. At first, I called this attitude a healthy egoism. Today I know it is "LOVE OF ONESELF."

As I began to love myself, I quit trying to always be right, and ever since I was wrong less of the time. Today I discovered, that is "MODESTY."

As I began to love myself, I refused to go on living in the past and worrying about the future. Now, I only live for the moment, where everything is happening. Today I live each day, day by day, and I call it "FULFILLMENT."

As I began to love myself, I recognized that my mind can disturb me and it can make me sick. But as I connected it to my heart, my mind became a valuable ally. Today I call this connection "WISDOM OF THE HEART."

We no longer need to fear arguments, confrontations or any kind of problems with ourselves or others. Even stars collide, and out of their crashing new worlds are born. Today I know "THAT IS LIFE

Now that we know how to care for and love ourselves everyday by entering the Physical, Intellectual, Emotional, and Spiritual rooms; let us seek to create a circle of women who will help us evolve into our next stanza.

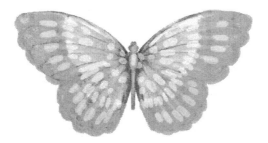

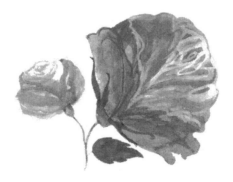

Author Photos

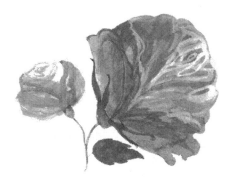

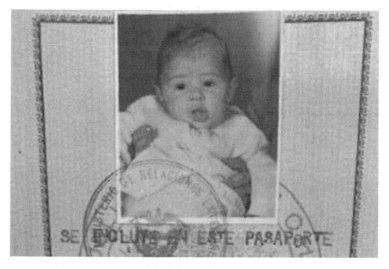

I finally arrive in NYC!

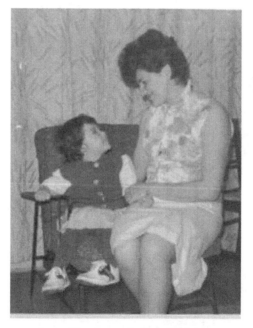

A mother's evolution into her
higher self benefits everyone

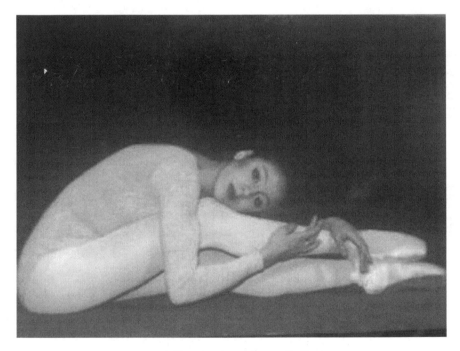

Dreaming of living abroad as a ballerina.

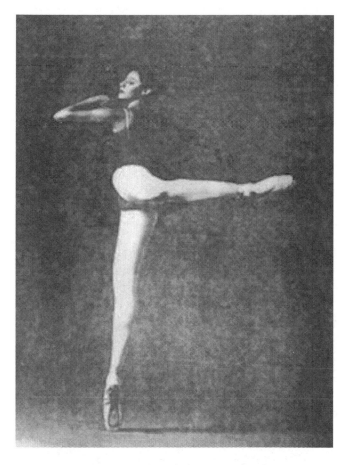

Windemere Ballet Theater Queens, NYC

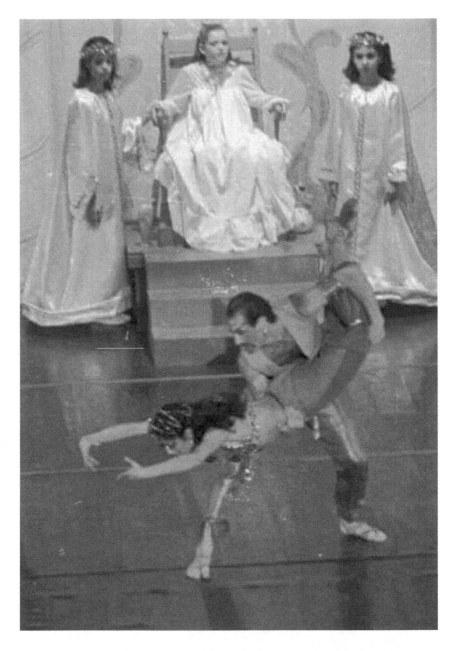

The Nutcracker, Arabian with amazing partner John Luther.

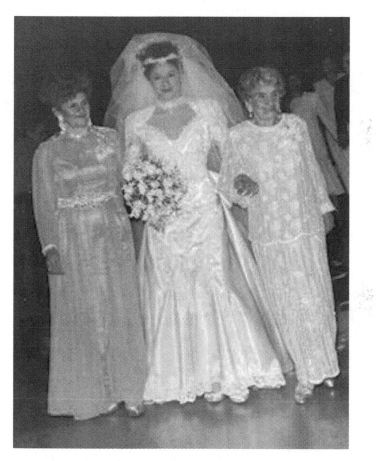

St. Patrick Cathedral on Fifth Ave allows the first mother
and grandmother to walk a bride down the aisle.

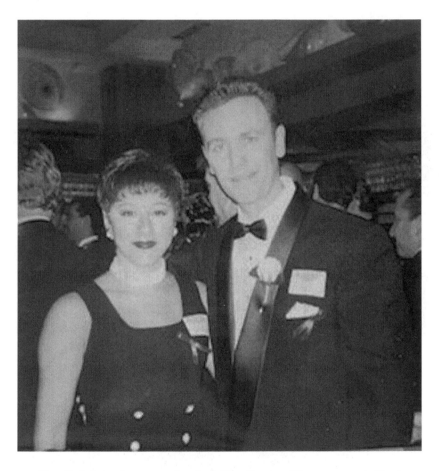

The Rainbow Room at Rockefeller Center. The answer is Yes!
Let's have a baby!

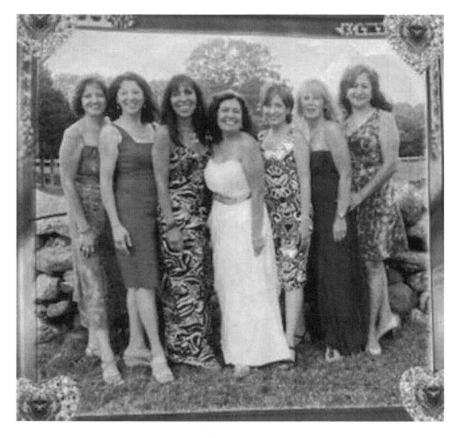

The benefit of friends. Celebrating 40 years of high school
sisterhood.

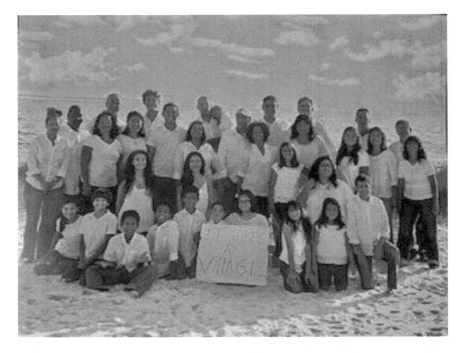

It Takes a village

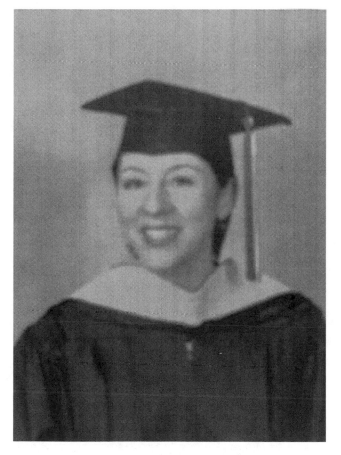

A happy graduate with a master's in
physical therapy.

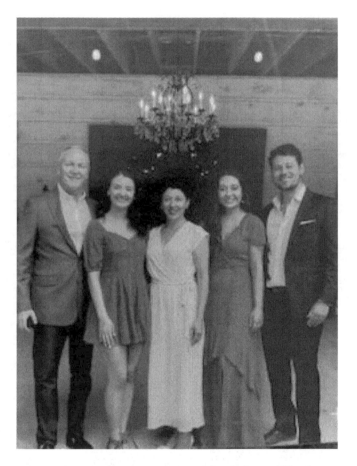

When a woman cares and loves herself her
whole family evolves with her.

Chapter Six:
The Benefits of Having Friends

Find Your Tribe

When I first arrived on the Gulf Coast of Mississippi, I felt extremely lonely. My definition of loneliness is a wolf without a pack or an indigenous person without a tribe/village. The odds of survival are low. Also, I personally feel it is one of the roots of physical, emotional, and spiritual pain. I had left my entire family and all my friends back in New York. I was a wolf without a pack, a woman without a tribe/village. I knew that I had to become part of a new pack/tribe/village of women. So, I started looking for a church affiliated women's group that would uplift me and provide a healthy environment for my family.

Little did I know that these women would be there for me through the good, the bad, and the ugly during the raising of our three children. In fact, I will even go so far as to say that I am still married for thirty years and our kids are still walking the earth because of these faith-filled, women-friends of Our Lady of Fatima church and the ACTS community. To be without a tribe is a choice.

Marriage

I remember one day; I had enough of my marriage and told my female church friends that I was done. One of them, instead of responding, just started telling a story of a woman back in South Africa that had a horrible husband. The husband went too far and crossed the line, though it was not physical abuse. She knew she could easily leave him, and no one would blame her. However, instead of leaving him, she made him his dinner and brought it to him like she always did. Her husband was shocked and after that day he started treating her with more love and kindness. This story made me think of my grandmother's story.

Carmen Maria Galindo, born in 1903 in Colombia, South America, married a man twenty years older than herself, and they had six children. The third child was a happy little boy, and at the age of five, he became sick. My grandmother was an herbalist, and familiar with the healing aspects of the body. Her husband wanted to take the boy out, but my grandmother told him not to because he was ill. He needed to stay home and heal. She told me, "I begged him to leave him home. It was much too cold outside." He dismissed her pleas and took him out.

When they returned the boy looked pale and very tired. The little boy became sicker every day after that. He never recovered, and days later, he died. My grandmother's pain and suffering turned into hatred. She hated her husband after that and couldn't bear to be near him. In her words, "He killed my little boy. My beautiful little son."

After months of mourning and anguish, she recognized forgiveness was the only way out of her severe hatred, misery, and life of hell. The woman she was closest to was the Virgin Mary. Her constant connection with the divine Mother was so deep you could almost say she channeled her. If she was to call herself devoted to The Virgin Mary, or the feminine Divine, who is only pure love, then there was no place for hatred within her. Mary told my grandmother to forgive her husband. There were five other children who needed the presence of a united mother and father.

She decided to start serving her husband dinner again. He had grown accustomed to her disdain and was also in severe grief and shame. When she gave him his dinner, he was shocked. He knew that what he never expected to occur had just happened. From that day forward, he never disagreed with my grandmother. In her words, "Our marriage did not return to how it was before, but with the Virgin Mary's guidance, I was able to go on." My grandmother was the first one to teach me that marriages depend on how many times a woman can forgive.

Women's stories like these must be told so our marriages can grow and evolve. It takes a village not only to raise a child, but to maintain marriages. Women have taught me to laugh, love, pray, and enjoy life despite all the unforeseeable circumstances which will always appear when we least expect them.

We all went to a marriage class together that year. I highly recommend Gary Chapman's, *The 5 Love Languages*. It's fantastic! Create your village. Create your tribe.

Girls' Night

After graduating from high school, my first tribe of six female friends and I went our separate ways. We attended different colleges and our careers and marriages took us away from each other. We did, however, manage to stay in touch. The year we all turned fifty, one of us remarried, and we all reunited for the first time at the wedding. When I say it was healing, it wouldn't be fully explaining the joy we felt to be together again. It turned into a Girls Night! Actually, it was a whole weekend of fun and laughter. We have been getting together almost every year since then and supporting each other on a group text. It's amazing how all of us have survived so much and remain so strong. We are continually evolving into our higher selves.

If you miss a friend from high school or college, call her today. Odds are she misses you, also. We women we are meant to be together. Why? Because we heal each other to the depths of our souls. Our feminine divine energy searches us out and unites us. Unfortunately, sometimes instead of seeking each other, we push each other away and seclude ourselves.

When your friend calls you, does this sound familiar? "Hi (your name) do you have time for lunch or dinner next week"? Your answer, "Oh I wish I could, but I have so much work to catch up on," or "My kids need me to go to their soccer practice." "My kids need me to go to their basketball practice." "My kids need me to go to their swimming practice" or "volleyball," or "tennis." And, "I have so much cleaning to do." You know this is you; come on admit it. You may be saying, "Being a social woman sounds wonderful, but who has the time"? "I have to cook dinner." "I have to do laundry." "I have to go food shopping; there is nothing in my fridge." "I want to watch Netflix." "I just want to get some sleep!"

Well, if you want to escape future doctor or therapist visits and prevent illnesses, get yourself some buddy time. Studies show that the brains of women who are out having fun with other women, create serotonin and oxytocin. These are the same hormones found in antidepressants. In the article, "The Healthy Benefits of A Girls' Night," it says, Meanwhile, . . . [t]he famed Harvard University Nurses' Health Study, which has studied women's health over a period of decades, concluded not having regular contact with girlfriends was as detrimental to her health as smoking or packing on pounds (Cooney)." In theory, if you want to lose weight and be healthy, it's time for Girls' Night.

Also, "In 2002, a landmark UCLA study concluded that girlfriends are stress-busters for women and have an impact on overall mood. It seems that when we're around friends, the mood-elevating hormone oxytocin is released, increasing our feelings of euphoria (Cooney)."

If you want to have less stress and be happier in your life, go have brunch with the girls! Hugging our sisters or anyone we care about also heals us.

Hugs Heal

I first learned the power of a hug from my four-year-old son. I remember I was in the kitchen washing dishes. I don't remember why, but I was crying. Maybe it had something to do with being a stay-at-home mom of three kids under the age of six, and it was the end of the day. Motherhood is the hardest career you'll ever experience, but worth every minute. All of a sudden, my little boy appeared in my peripheral vision. As I turned to see what he needed, he looked up at me and just wrapped his tiny arms around my legs and hugged me. That hug was so powerfully healing, I instantly felt all the love in the universe come into my legs and up into the rest of my body. This child felt so much compassion; he instinctively knew what to do. I stopped crying of course. And I bent down and hugged him back. I definitely felt better after that hug. The recollection brings tears to my eyes. His hug made me a hugger for life.

Virginia Satir was one of the first psychotherapists and family therapists to speak about the importance of hugs and physical touch. She is well known for the quantifying of daily hugs:

- *We need four hugs a day for survival,*
- *We need eight hugs a day for maintenance,*
- *We need twelve hugs a day for growth*

Hugs Change Our Biochemistry

Hugging releases dopamine, which controls the brain's reward and pleasure centers and serotonin, which we've learned regulates mood, appetite, digestion, sleep, sexual desire, and social behavior. It also releases endorphins, natural pain and stress fighters, and oxytocin, the love or cuddle hormone, which reduces your levels of stress hormones cortisol and adrenaline. When stress goes down, your immune system, located mostly in your gut, works better. The pressure of a hug may stimulate the thymus gland, which is responsible for the regulation and balance of white blood cells that protect us from infections and foreign invaders. Less stress also lowers your heart rate and blood pressure, which may reduce potential risk for heart disease.

Zen Master Thich Nhat Hanh, who made hugging meditation famous, is a global thought leader whose key teaching is that through mindfulness, people can learn to live in the present moment. He believes a good hug may have life-changing effects on the individual. He writes about his pursuit of hugging meditation:

"When we hug, our hearts connect, and we know that we are not separate beings. Hugging with mindfulness and concentration can bring reconciliation, healing, understanding, and much happiness. You can practice hugging meditation with a friend, a child, your parents, or even a tree. To practice, first bow to each other and recognize each other's presence. Then, enjoy three deep, conscious breaths to bring yourself fully into the present moment. Next, open your arms and begin hugging, holding each other for three in-and-out-breaths. With the first breath, become aware that you are present in this very moment and feel happy. With the second breath, become aware that the other person is present in this moment and feel happy as well. With the third breath, become aware that you are here together, right now on this Earth. We can feel deep gratitude and happiness for our togetherness. Finally, release the other person and bow to each other to show your thanks (Hanh).

A good time for a hugging meditation is when your kids leave, and the house is empty.

Embracing the Empty Nest

One of the major life-changing, evolving events in a mother's or father's life is the empty nest, I first noticed it when I ran into a middle-aged friend at the grocery store. I asked her how she was doing, and she said, "I am not doing too well with this empty nest thing. Both my daughters are out of my house, and I don't like it. I am really not handling it well." This felt to me like she was lost. I was feeling her sadness and her displacement. This reminded me of when I was lost and evolving out of my "dancer" identity. She was evolving out of her "caregiver mother" identity. I felt really bad for her and recommended she get together with her

115

friends and become a volunteer so she could focus on caring for others who really needed her.

Flash forward to the year my last child graduated from high school. All was well until I was climbing into bed one night and noticed a tremendous sense of quiet in the house, like someone had died. Then all of a sudden, I had a vision that my son was touching my hand. He was about eight and he said, "Mom, can I climb in bed with you?"

My response was, "Of course you can, my love, you don't have to ask." My heart stopped and I felt as if I was in mourning. I began to cry. I texted my son, now twenty and in the military, and told him what happened. He was fine and said, "I love you mom." Well, if he was okay, what was going on with me? I cried myself to sleep. For the next forty-eight hours, I was miserable. My heart was broken.

I wrote in my journal, "Lord, I am experiencing the intense sorrow of the passing of my kids' childhoods, the death of being a mom of young kids and teenagers. I feel ashamed of my emotions because my kids are not dead. They're perfectly fine, well-adjusted young adults." "My heart is tearing apart. I am dying." "Where did the time go"? "I am mourning the death of a part of me as 'Mother.'" "It is the end of an era. The past is gone." The next morning, I went to yoga. Tears fell on the yoga mat like drops of rain. Intense body pain left my body as energy and water. I lay on the mat and started doing EFT; "Even though I feel intense sorrow, loss, and anxiety, I deeply love and accept myself. I am healing."

When I got home, I started self-treating, myofascial release. I applied pressure to my psoas muscles, which are metaphysically considered the emotional muscles because they often hold on to trauma. I cried some more and felt my intense pain. I was leaving the care-giving stage and evolving into my next stanza of my life, the "Back to Me" stanza.

How Can You Evolve from Empty Nest Syndrome? If you're feeling a sense of loss;

- Feel all your emotions. Yes, you can cry! You can climb into bed and pull the covers over your head.
- Write in a journal and put down your raw heartfelt feelings. Anything you keep to yourself may affect you physically. Let it go!
- Talk to women you feel will be understanding. Not all women experience empty nest syndrome. Those who have will share their experience with you and be more compassionate. Avoid people who usually say, "Just be strong" or "That's life, that's how it is."
- If you feel it's overwhelming, then speak to a counselor or talk to a therapist sooner rather than later.
- Start buying cards you can send your daughter or son every week to make them smile; chances are they will get homesick and miss you, too.
- Create care packages they will love to receive.
- Join a youth group that always needs adults to provide food or support.
- Start date nights with your spouse. If you are single, create time for a girls' night.
- Give yourself permission to explore this new life. You have more freedom and more time. What are your interests or hobbies? It's time to find out what you love.
- Walk around the house naked! Why? Because now you can. You have evolved into the new YOU!
- Accept that you will always be Mom. No matter how far they roam, they will always be your kids.

- Praise your daughter or son for their independence and their courage. Let them know you are their number one cheerleader.

It's good to make new friends, especially when we're empty nesting, but the relationships that we already have may need some healing. Why? because they can create physical pain.

Can relationship problems cause pain in your body?

The simple answer is, "Heck yeah!" I remember the first time I knew for sure that our emotions from our relationships create pain in the body. I was treating a nurse for pain in her buttock. After three treatments her pain went away. Then it came back the following month. During her treatment I asked her if there had been any stress occurring at work or at home because sometimes emotions can create fascial restrictions. Her eyes got wide and she said, "Oh my gosh, I had an argument with my husband last month before I came to see you and we just had another argument again yesterday. My husband is the pain in my butt!" We both laughed out loud, but we also knew there was truth in this statement.

Fascia, our connective tissue, doesn't just respond to a physical problem, but also to emotional and spiritual difficulties. Next time you're having an argument with a family member, friend, or co-worker be aware of what your body does. You may notice rapid breathing, a tight jaw/belly/buttock, you can't poop, shoulders may go up, neck starts to hurt, your throat gets tight, a headache begins, your body becomes warm; all of these are fascial restrictions.

What's Happening? Your thoughts are sending messages to your cells that something is very wrong. The fascia is part of your cells' membrane and so the connective tissue/fascia starts to tighten up. Muscles which are made of fascia lock up. The environment of your cells, muscles, has now changed from loose and peaceful which is how you felt a few seconds ago, to a hostile environment also called the fight/flight/freeze response.

The 3 things that help my body decrease pain during relationship problems are:

1. Quiet the mind- I excuse myself and just say, "I'll be back in a few minutes when I am calmer." Sit in silence and take deep breaths for 5 min or more to allow my mind to stop figuring things out. If you want to be in a place of peace, you must create peace. For me it's just sitting quietly and being with God. Wish I knew this when I was raising three kids!

2. Don't take anything personally- the other person's words and actions were causing me physical, emotional and spiritual pain because I allowed it. I don't allow it anymore. A book that I love that taught me this is, *The Four Agreements,* by Miguel Ruiz.

3. Put myself in their shoes. If it's my mother I try to see it from her perspective. She is getting older, set in her ways, and patience may not be her virtue. She also still feels she needs to protect me from the world because she will always be my mom. If it's my children, I must see the world through their eyes. They can do this on their own and listening to me is not on their agenda. A parent's experience is not always what they're interested in; It sure wasn't on my agenda when I was their age. When it's my husband I need to see his point of view which is always from the perspective of security and safety. Finance issues are the number one reason marriages don't last. If you see your husband as a caveman, then

it's easier to see his perspective. He needs to keep a roof over our family's heads and keep everyone fed and safe. Spending what we don't have or taking out from savings is not what cavemen like. Cavemen like to know that they are strong and needed. Belittling them destroys their soul. If you're waiting for them to share their emotions, you will have to wait till the next ice age. For me, my husband is the head (compromise is crucial) and I am the heart of our family.

Lastly, letting go of the need to be right with anyone, is a great way to decrease relationship problems and heal the pain in your body. Try it.

Science is Great, But How Can I Apply it?

Find your tribe. If you have no friends, make new friends. Join faith groups. Volunteer in community/hospital service groups, or businesswomen's groups. Join a yoga studio, a book club, a social justice group, or a theater group. Join the League of Women Voters, a garden club, a coffee group, the local chamber of commerce, or take art or cooking classes. The list is endless but choose what sparks your interest. What do you love? Work on your marriage. If we work on our marriages as much as we focus on our jobs eight hours a day, imagine how much money we'll save on therapy and divorce. Girls' Night and twelve hugs a day are life changing, simple, and fun. Healing our relationship problems by quieting our minds, not taking anything personally, putting ourselves in others' shoes, and letting go of the need to be right heals us. If we are to continue providing economic, spiritual, and social stability for everyone, then let's decrease our stress levels so we can continue the good work. Because ultimately, girls just want to have fun.

That's all we really want.

Chapter Seven:
Your New Place Each Time You Evolve

Evolving Ain't Easy

"The comfort zone is the great enemy to creativity; moving beyond it necessitates intuition, which in turn configures new perspectives and conquers fears."

--Dan Stevens

"We cannot become what we need to be by remaining what we are."

–Max dePree

Biloxi, Mississippi in 1995 was not the big, fun city it is now. It was a quiet, beautiful shrimping town on the Gulf Coast. The transition from New York City to Biloxi, as you may expect, was pretty tough. Women friends from church and the La Leche League kept me thriving. We had our second child in 1996, and at 36, I realized I needed to go back to school.

Somewhere in my heart I had held onto my dream of becoming a physical therapist, since I was nineteen. But wait a minute, "I am not smart enough and I am not good enough," I wrote in my journal one summer morning. I remember this vividly as I sat outside in Mary Mahone's Cafe. Then the next line was a flow of my pen. What I mean is my pen just kept writing. God answered, "How do you know if you don't try?" I responded, "Because I hate school, I hate studying, and I'm not a good student." "Why don't you just take one course?" A dialogue was occurring; that had never happened before! Something crazy was happening. Something inside of me started to sparkle like a firecracker, just like when I was nineteen in front of my first physical therapist, Abby. I decided at that very moment to feel the fear, jump into unknown territory, and get out of my comfort zone. As I always say, "Feel the fear and do it anyway!"

The nearest college was the University of South Alabama, an hour's drive away in Mobile. There I was told that my degree had essentially expired, and I would have to take about seven courses--and get A's in all of them--before they would even consider me as an applicant for the Master of Physical Therapy program. In shock and dismay, I went home and wrote in my journal, "God, what the heck was that all about?"

God responded, "What? You're going to let these little obstacles get in the way?"

Me: "You're calling seven courses all with A's little obstacles?" And whoever heard of an expiration on your college degree?

He replied, "Just take one of those courses and see how you do. Dip your toes into the water." Visualizing this I thought, well dipping my "toe in" means I don't have to put my whole foot in, I can quickly take it out. If I take one course, I will probably not like it, not do very well and then I can tell God, "I'm out." and not feel guilty. And so, it began.

Off I went to Biloxi's Jefferson Davis Community College with my paperwork from the university, and they all but laughed and said, " You can't take these courses until you take these math, science, and English classes, or you won't get A's in your chemistry, physics, anatomy and physiology classes." Fourteen classes! Are you kidding me? Remembering the whole dipping the toe thing, I put my newborn in the stroller, left my two-year-old at home with Papa, and headed to register with eighteen to twenty-five-year-old students at the community college.

I took a psychology course (This is where I learned about the nun study in Chapter Three), loved it, and got an A. Then it dawned on me, I WAS smart enough and good enough. Que the arch angels' heavenly voices!

I began to evolve into my next stanza and kept taking a class or two each semester. Oh yes, God threw in one more surprise, a third baby, a girl, in 1998. If you are open to divine wisdom and let go of control, magic happens. I never stopped breastfeeding. The community college even let me pump milk in their tutor's office. I received A's in everything except Physics I and II; I was grateful to receive B's.

I went for my interview in 2001 at the University of South Alabama with a 4.0 GPA. They were surprised to see me back. They then said, "Good job, Jackie. You just have to take the GRE, Graduate Record Exam, get a score of 1000, and then pass an interview with our school." This is where you can easily use expletives as a writer, but I'm sure you can use your imagination. I received a score of 850 on the GRE and wrote in my journal, "God, what is happening? I've done everything you told me to, birthed and breastfed three kids, and kept my marriage intact! I went back to college and got a 4.0. Why can't I get a higher score on the GRE? God says, "This is another little obstacle. Try again. I never said it would be easy." I took it again and scored high enough to get an interview. The interview was nerve-wracking. As the clinician held up my letter titled, "'Why I should be accepted into PT school'", another torturous requirement, he said, "We love the part in your letter where you say the reason you should be accepted into physical therapy school is because you inherited the PT gene from your grandmother. That's a new one. We've heard all the reasons, but this is hilarious.

I looked at them with a straight face and just said, "It's true. My grandmother Carmen was the only person in her Colombian village in the 1920s to help people with broken bones, sprains, hip and back pain, headaches, etc. She was called La Sobandera. I am like my grandmother. She taught me everything. I have been doing manual treatments for all of my dance and non-dance friends since I was fifteen." Their jaws dropped.

I received my acceptance letter soon after. By a miracle, I graduated with a master's degree in physical therapy from the University of South Alabama in 2004. Thank you Dr. Fell, Dr. Dale, Dr. Grey, Dr. Irion, Dr. Wall, and Dr. Jefferson. Little did I know the most difficult time in my life would be after I evolved into the next stanza.

The year from hell began. I found out there was something worse than not walking; I couldn't pass my PT licensing exam. As I watched all my classmates pass their licensure in their first or second try, I still couldn't pass. After my third inability to pass the test, my friends, Sharon Larose and Jule Miller, both psychiatrists, said I had test anxiety and recommended I get tested by a trained psychologist, Peter

Herring. Low and behold, they were right. After several sessions with Peter, I was able to pass my licensing exam on my next and final try. One thing my mom taught me was, "Never give up!"

From May 2004 to July 2005, I was not allowed to work as a PT, so no income was coming in. My husband had also injured his back from working long hours on roofs, so there was no income coming in from either of us.

I remember one time going to the store and having twenty-eight dollars to feed my family of five for one week. I bought rice and beans, pasta, ramen noodles, tuna fish, bread, milk and eggs. There are no words to describe to you what it is like to have zero income for a year for a family of five. What I will say--through the gut-wrenching pit of my stomach I am feeling right now and the tears that are rising and forming not letting me see these typed letters very clearly--is that no one ever said life would be easy. We all have our crosses to bear. So please be aware of anyone who does not have a lot of food in their shopping cart at the grocery store, but they have kids in tow. It's not always because they just came in for a few things; it may be that they do not have enough money to feed their families.

This experience has made me stronger and more compassionate. When in the grocery store, I see a parent fitting this description, I quickly buy a gift card at the cash register and then find the mom or dad in the aisle and give it to them with a smile and walk away. No words exchanged just a simple knowing during eye contact. Pain and suffering create compassion and makes us one.

During this year of misery, I remember saying, Lord, help me to stay healthy so I don't literally have a heart attack from this severe stress and die. I decided right then and there I was

125

going to care and love myself. This is when my daily ritual of health began. I woke up at 6:00 A.M. to practice yoga and meditate for 30 minutes. At 6:30 get kids dressed and fed. At 7:00 put Alyssa and Logan on the school bus. Bathe myself and get dressed. At 7:45 drive Sofia to school. At 8:15 walk on the school walking track for 45 minutes. Head to Barnes and Noble for six hours to study for my next PT exam. Then at 3:00 P.M. pick up Sofia from school, head home for afternoon tea with kids: cook, help with homework, dance, soccer, or whatever else was going on each day. I remembered to have fun, laugh, write in my gratitude journal, and stay focused on all the good that was happening all around me. Scott's back healed and he began to get handyman jobs. Our family and friends were a great help.

On July 15th, 2005 I walked to the mailbox. I did this everyday a couple of weeks after my PT exams. I opened the letter from the MS Board of Physical Therapy, and it said, "We are happy to inform you that you have passed your PT exam for licensure." My whole body froze; then I broke down. I literally fell to the floor. All I kept on saying was "Thank you Lord!" as I lay my hands on the floor and sobbed. I got up and ran to the house with outbursts of, "I passed my exam." Scott and the kids were so happy that their faces revealed to me what a burden this had been for them as well. I then went to bed to be grateful and sob some more. It was over. The hell was over.

Just as it may not be comfortable for the caterpillar to lay in the cocoon until she becomes a beautiful butterfly, neither is it easy to evolve into each stanza of our lives. Our bodies, careers, and family life change: our hormones fluctuate, we can't pass our exams, we lose our jobs, divorce happens, lumps grow, organs start faltering, car accidents occur, teeth get infected, jaws lock down, snoring begins, parents become ill, we become adult caregivers, family members die, kids go astray. I need to stop because I can see the look on your face. No one prepared us for this. So, what do we do? We ask some questions.

In *Women Who Run with The Wolves*, Clarissa Pinkola Estes, PhD, tells us, "Asking the proper question is the central action of transformation-in fairy tales, in analysis, and in individuation. The key question causes germination of consciousness. The properly shaped question always emanates from an essential curiosity about what stands behind. Questions are the keys which cause the secret doors of the psyche to swing open (Estes, 52)."

What questions do we need to ask ourselves when we are stuck, sick of being sick and tired, unemployed, or burned out? What questions will swing the four doors in our house open so we can evolve into our next stanza no matter our health, finances, or presumed lack of time?

1. What do I love and what makes me feel joy?

2. What do I visualize myself being or doing?

3. What are my fears?

4. Am I worthy of my dream?

Write the answers down and look at your words. If you are uncomfortable and afraid; then you have done a good job. Create your ritual of Self Care/Self Love. Go and open the four P.I.E.S. Connect with the high vibrational frequency of love, and this will carry you to the next creative stanza of your life.

"Life isn't about finding yourself. Life is about creating yourself (Top)." George Bernard Shaw

Creativity

During the year I was at the skilled nursing facility after hurricane Katrina, a therapist recommended that I take a class in manual training with John F. Barnes, PT. I remember my professor at PT school recommended that we all study the fascial system and mentioned Barnes's name. I was curious because I had some right side back pain from a previous injury lifting a patient, so I decided to check it out to see if his class could help me with this pain. My first Myofascial release class was nothing short of life changing. It was as if everything John said for those three days was a return to my grandmother's treatments. "Don't be afraid to place your hands on your patients with gentle sustained pressure, never force, listen, and don't rush, connect and be with your patients. Trust the work and do the work." I returned from that class with a new purpose in life, and I knew I was evolving and creating a new life.

Treating my patients with Myofascial Release was so loving that I knew I needed to share it with the other therapists in the skilled nursing facility. I conducted an in-service training and introduced everyone on staff to John F. Barnes, MFR. I soon realized it would be difficult to spend time with my patients and do this healing work. In an institutional setting there is nothing slow about physical therapy, and unfortunately, we don't always get time to just be with our patients. Time is money and productivity is important. There are always other patients in the waiting room. Unfortunately, paperwork also occupies much of a therapist's time, so I quickly realized after one year that I needed to find another venue that would allow me more time with my patients. I evolved into an outpatient PT at a hospital.

I was hired by Ken Ackerman as a John F. Barnes myofascial release PT for Gulf Coast Physical Therapy in Gulfport, Mississippi. This role allowed me to spend additional time with more involved patients suffering from stroke, TMJ, severe migraines, fibromyalgia, and even patients in comas. I loved it! It was also my first time working in another part of the hospital where they had a psychiatric unit. These patients suffering from depression and many other issues loved to be touched, and their connection to their mind, body, and spirit pain was evident. Their beautiful loving words after I treated them brought me to an awareness that something else was happening there, and it had to do with the fascial system. Our bodies hold onto painful memories and trauma; these are often expressed as physical pain by restricting the fascial system, as noted in the book *Healing Ancient Wounds* by John F. Barnes (Barnes,).

Working in outpatient, ICU, inpatient, and the psych unit was hard on my body, but I learned to leave the building for my hour-long lunch break, sit in the sun, and walk on a walking track for twenty to thirty minutes before I came home. Sadly, after a year, I thought when Ken called me into the office, he would be giving me a raise, but instead he said, "Jackie, since Hurricane Katrina, the hospital has not done very well and is closing, so our contract is up. I am sorry, but we are letting you and others go." Right then, God's voice in my head said, "Time to fly, little butterfly." I believe this was code for, "Your butt is evolving again."

I had already been treating patients on Thursday afternoons at the River Rock Yoga studio in Ocean Springs, thanks to Moira Anderson, so I simply said, "Don't worry guys, I will be fine. I will just start my own full-time practice." They immediately replied, "You won't last six months because you won't take insurance. Go and interview

129

with these other hospitals and they will hire you." Luckily, I followed Gods plan instead. I'm grateful to have celebrated the twelfth-year anniversary in October 2019 of my healing space called, Gulf Coast Myofascial Release Physical Therapy, in Ocean Springs. I have John F. Barnes to thank for that: align with your essence to find your life's purpose.

Many people will not want you to evolve into your next stanza, my friends, but your passion, your truth, and your perseverance will change their minds, and doors will open!

Evolve and re-create yourself. Every stanza and space of your life is important, but what keeps it moving forward is your creativity. It's what feeds your evolution. It's what the world needs. Dr. Christiane Northrup puts it this way,

"The world needs a lot of creativity right now if we are going to solve our problems, and it yearns for the wisdom of seasoned women who own their Goddess nature. We're entering a new age of experience and bringing back the sacred feminine energy, also known as yin or the female principle, which was central to the lives and beliefs of humanity for the vast majority of prehistory. The sacred feminine influenced the rituals, ceremonies, religions, myths, legends and artwork, of ancient civilizations all around the world for thousands and thousands of years---far longer than the relatively new era of written history, which is a mere blip on the screen. And according to many anthropologists, the sacred feminine was worshiped as a Great Goddess or Mother Earth. It's definitely time to bring Mama back (Northrop, 19)."

Another woman I greatly admire has touched the core of my belief systems. If we are to evolve as women, we cannot do it in a vacuum. What is occurring to our earth, our government, and the countries of the world has a role to play in our health.

I now introduce you to Sister Joan.

What Occurs Around Us Affects Us

Sister Joan D. Chittister, O.S.B., is an American Benedictine nun, theologian, author, and speaker. She has served as prioress and Benedictine federation president, president of the Leadership Conference of Women Religious, and co-chair of the Global Peace Initiative of Women. Sister Joan has written fifty books on peace, justice, and equality. Her latest one is called, *The Time Is Now; A Call to Uncommon Courage.* Here is an excerpt:

"The future depends on whether we make serious decisions about our own roles in shaping a future that fulfills God's will for the world, or we simply choose to suffer the decisions made by others intent on imposing their own vision of tomorrow. This moment is a daunting one. At every crossroad, every one of us has three possible options. The first choice is to quit a road going somewhere we do not want to go. We can move on in another direction. We can distance ourselves from the difficulties of it all. We can leave the mission unfinished.

The second alternative is to crawl into a comfortable cave with nice people and become a church, a culture, a society within a society. We can just hunker down together and wait for the storm to calm down, go by, and become again the nice warm womb of our beginnings. The third choice is to refuse to accept a moral deterioration of the present and insist on celebrating the coming of an unknown, but surely holier, future. (Chittister,)."

Now you're probably asking, why did you have to go there? I don't have to make any choices. I don't need more problems to worry about. Trust me, I understand. But, I'm not being honest if I don't include that ignoring what is occurring to our earth, government, and other countries won't affect us, because it already does. The unhealthy food we eat, the air we breathe, the divisiveness of our political parties, and our lack of compassion for the people who are oppressed in our country and other nations *does* affect our health. Our environment does affect our cells/genes. Maybe what we really need is to remove fear and allow ourselves to change in order to evolve into our higher selves.

In her book *Outrageous Openness,* Tosha Silver leads us into our next stanza with a poem:

CHANGE ME PRAYER

"Divine Beloved, Change Me into someone

who can give with complete ease and abundance,

knowing You are the unlimited Source of All.

Let me be an easy open conduit for Your prosperity.

Let me trust that all of my own needs are

always met in amazing ways

and it is safe to give freely as my heart guides me.

And equally, please Change Me into someone

who can feel wildly open to receiving.

Let me know my own value, beauty and

worthiness without question.

Let me allow others the supreme pleasure of giving to me.

Let me feel worthy to receive in every possible way.

And let me extend kindness to all who need,

feeling compassion and understanding

in even the hardest situations.

Change me into One who can fully love, forgive and accept myself

so I may carry your Light without restriction.

Let everything that needs to go, go.

Let everything that needs to come, come.

I am utterly Your own.

You are Me.

I am You.

We are One.

All is well (Silver).

***

What Do We Do Now?

I truly believe that to evolve we must first care and love this temple, this body/mind/spirit. As we let go of what needs to go, we make space for what needs to come. Visiting each room of our house each day, the physical, intellectual, emotional, and spiritual keeps us connected to God, right side of the brain, Inner wisdom, Source, Higher Self, Universe, Light, Holy Spirit, Intuition, or Inner Voice. This is where the magic happens. This is where we evolve and take our first step out of the cocoon into our next creative stanza.

On the following pages I share with you a simple worksheet that I give my patients for what needs to come. I've filled out the first page as an example of choices for my own house with four rooms. I look at this sheet every day.

The latter pages are blank for you to fill out with your choices for your own house. Write as many options for each room that you enjoy. Copy it and place it on your bathroom mirror, refrigerator, and workspace. Look at it every day to create your habit of Self-Care/Self-Love.

A HOUSE WITH FOUR ROOMS

I am Jackie Castro-Cooper. My identity isn't the work that I do or the career that I've chosen. My identity is to honor myself as a divine spiritual being. The amount of love that I give to myself expands into everyone around me and into the world. The more love I fill myself with, the more love my family, friends, community, and country will receive. I am open to my creativity, which is divinely inspired. This short human experience on this earth is a gift. This human body, my temple, in which my spirit lives is also a gift. From today forward I will see my body as a house/temple with four rooms. Each day I will open each room and choose something from each room as a caring, loving gift to myself.

PHYSICAL

- *Walk along the trees*
- *stroll on the beach*
- *hike in the mountains*
- *dance in my living room*
- *morning yoga at home*
- *yoga before bed*
- *Zumba class/ or yoga class*
- *go to the gym for strength training or the treadmill*

INTELLECTUAL

- *My thoughts are energy.*
- *I choose to believe that I can heal myself therefore the environment of my cells/genes receive the message to do the work of healing.*
- *I look in the mirror every morning and smile.*

• I read inspirational books when I take a bath in the morning that create thoughts of optimism, laughter, and gratitude.

• I learn something new every day to awaken dormant neurons.

EMOTIONAL

Write in my journal for 15 minutes.

- *What emotions am I feeling?*

- *What do I need to tell someone?*

- *What do I need?*

- *Laugh out loud*

- *Cry into a pillow*

- *Scream in the car*

- *Where can I put the four-inch ball to release my fascia? Where am I stiff?*

- *Where do I feel physical pain?*

- *I allow myself to feel my emotions in a yoga class*

- *Tap (EFT) for 15 minutes to decrease my negative emotions.*

SPIRITUAL

Slow deep breaths x 10 reps

Meditate for 1, 5, 10, 20 min,

Raise my thoughts to peace, love, joy, oneness, God

Pray, church

A HOUSE WITH FOUR ROOMS

I am_____ (your name), my identity isn't the work that I do or the career that I've chosen. My identity is to honor myself as a divine spiritual being. The amount of love that I give to myself expands into everyone around me and into the world. The more love I fill myself with, the more love my family, friends, community, and country will receive. I am open to my creativity, which is divinely inspired. This short human experience on this earth is a gift. This human body, my temple, in which my spirit lives is also a gift. From today forward I will see my body as a house/temple with four rooms. Each day I will open each room and choose something from each room as a caring, loving gift to myself.

PHYSICAL

-
-
-
-
-
-

INTELLECTUAL

-
-
-
-
-
-

EMOTIONAL

-
-
-

-
-
-

SPIRITUAL

-
-
-
-
-
-

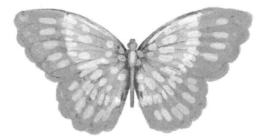

Epilogue

My Friends,

It's been a life changing experience writing this book. It's ten years of my own evolution into the power of the self-care/self-love movement. I'm not the same person I was before delving into my past and the research that created the book you now hold in your hands. I have discovered wisdom that I would never have discovered if I hadn't gone in search of the truth. It's made me a better person. This book has been a labor of love. May you always remember what my mother and grandmother said, "Your body, mind, and spirit are holy. Treat them as such," and "Joy comes only from you, who creates it."

I leave you in the palms of God's hands as you read one of my very favorite quotes from the book, *A Return to Love, A Course in Miracles.*

"Our Deepest fear is not that we are inadequate.

Our deepest fear is that we are powerful beyond measure.

It is our light, not our darkness that most frightens us.

We ask ourselves, who am I to be brilliant, gorgeous, talented, and fabulous?

Actually, who are you not to be?

You are a child of God.

Your playing small doesn't serve the world. There's nothing enlightened about shrinking

So that other people won't feel insecure around you.

We were born to make manifest the Glory of God that is within us.

It's not just in some of us; it's in everyone.

And as we let our own light shine, we unconsciously give other people

Permission to do the same.

As we are liberated from our own fear,

our presence automatically liberates others."
Mary Ann Williamson

With love and health,

Jackie Castro Cooper

About The Author

Jackie Castro-Cooper, MPT received her master's in physical therapy at the age of forty, with her three small children and 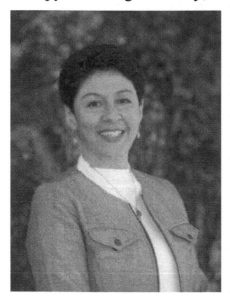 husband at her side. After working in hospitals, acute, subacute, outpatient, skilled nursing facilities and nursing homes, Jackie decided to open her own practice. Despite the odds she opened up the first holistic, integrative practice in Mississippi, Gulf Coast Myofascial Release Physical Therapy in 2007, and for over 12 years continues to provide care for chronic pain sufferers, women's health issues, internal pelvic work, intraoral TMJ, babies and children's health issues.

Jackie's personal experience with physical pain from a twelve year career in ballet and musical theater, coupled with life experiences of not being able to walk after giving birth, burnout, and dealing with a feeling of not being smart or good enough to be a wife, mom, and a physical therapist have colored her life during her own evolutions.

www.gcmfr.com

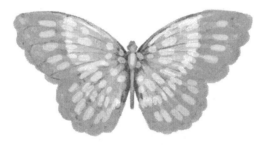

Works Cited

"6 Personality Traits Associated with Longevity." *Awaken*, 6 July 2012, www.awaken.com/2012/07/6-personality-traits-associated-with-longevity/.

"7 Fascinating Scientific Findings of Meditating Monks' Brains." *EOC Institute*, eocinstitute.org/meditation/buddhist-monk-meditation-2/.

"Academy of Iridology." *Academy of Iridology*, www.iridologyacademy.org/.

"A Quote by Charlie Chaplin." *Goodreads*, Goodreads, www.goodreads.com/quotes /809976-as-i-that-anguish.

Alschuler, Lise. "The HPA Axis." *Integrative Therapeutics, LLC*, 31 Oct. 2016, www.integrativepro.com/Resources/Integrative-Blog/2016/The-HPA-Axis.

Agnvall, Elizabeth. "Stress and Disease - Conditions That May Be Caused by Chronic Stress." *AARP*, 1 Nov. 2014, www.aarp.org/health/healthy-living/info-2014/ stress-and-disease.html.

Barnes, John F. *Myofascial Release: Healing Ancient Wounds: The Renegades Wisdom*. Rehabilitation Services, Inc., T/A MFR Treatment Centers & Seminars, 2016.

Barnes, John F. "Advance Your Myofascial Release Skills." *Myofascial Release Treatment Centers & Seminars*, www.myofascialrelease.com/downloads

"Benedictine Monk, Brother David Steindl-Rast on How to Have Faith during Difficult Times." *Facebook Watch*, www.facebook.com/SuperSoulSunday/videos/15338405433 30127/.

"Benefits of Yoga." *American Osteopathic Association*, www.osteopathic.org/what-is-osteopathic-medicine/benefits-of-yoga/.

"Bienvenid@s a La Risoterapia Con Mari Cruz García Rodera." *Mari Cruz García Rodera*, www.maricruzgarcia.com/.

Boccio, Frank Jude. "Q&A: How Are Relaxation and Meditation Different?" *Yoga Journal*, 3 June 2008, www.yogajournal.com/meditation/relaxation-vs-meditation.

Boehm, Julia K., PhD. "Relation Between Optimism and Lipids in Midlife." https://doi.org/10.1016/j.amjcard.2013.01.292, 25 February 2013.

Brogan, Kelly, and Kristen Loberg. *A Mind of Your Own, The Truth About Depression and How Women Can Heal Their Bodies to Reclaim Their Lives*. Harperwave, 2017.

Brogan, Kelly. "Flipping the Script on Menopause: Dr. Christiane Northrup." *Kelly Brogan MD*, 16 Aug. 2017, www.kellybroganmd.com/flipping-the-script-on-menopause-dr-christiane- northrup/.

Burch, Vidyamala, and Danny Penman. *You Are Not Your Pain: Using Mindfulness to Relieve Pain, Reduce*

Stress, and Restore Well-Being---an Eight-Week Program. Flatiron Books, 2015.

Cavill, Nick, Kahleier, Sonja, and Racioppi, Francesca, eds. "Physical activity and health in Europe: Evidence for action," World Health Organization: Europe. www.euro.who.int/data/assets/pdf_file/0011/87545/E89490.pdf

Chang, Yu-Kai, et al. "Effect of Resistance-Exercise Training on Cognitive Function in Healthy Older Adults: a Review." *Journal of Aging and Physical Activity,* Centre for Reviews and Dissemination (UK), Oct. 2012, www.ncbi.nlm.nih.gov/pubmed/22186664.

Chittister, Joan. *The Time Is Now: A Call to Uncommon Courage.* Convergent, 2019.

Chopra, Deepak, et al. "Deepak Explains the Deeper Meaning of Yoga." *The Chopra Center,* 24 Aug. 2016, www.chopra.com/articles/deepak-explains-the-deeper-meaning-of-yoga.

Church, Dawson. *The Genie in Your Genes: Epigenetic Medicine and the New Biology of Intention.* Energy Psychology Press, 2014.

Church, Dawson. "Tap Your Way to Healing With EFT." *Omega,* 10 June 2019, www.eomega.org/article/tap-your-way-to-healing-with-eft.

Cooney, Beth. "The Healthy Benefits of a Girls Night." *Connecticut Post,* Healthy Life, 9 May 2011, www.ctpost.com/healthyyou/spirit/article/The-Healthy-Benefits-of-a-Girls-Night-1351362.php.

Cousins N. Anatomy of an Illness as Perceived by the Patient. New England Journal of Medicine. 1976; 295(26):1458–63

"Dan Stevens Quotes." *BrainyQuote*, Xplore, www.brainyquote.com/quotes/dan_stevens_492332.

"David R. Hawkins Quote." *A*, www.azquotes.com/quote/1033689.

Davis, Carol M. *Integrative Therapies in Rehabilitation: Evidence for Efficacy in Therapy, Prevention, and Wellness.* SLACK Incorporated, 2017.

Dinan, Timothy G, and John F Cryan. "Microbes, Immunity, and Behavior: Psychoneuroimmunology Meets the Microbiome." *Neuropsychopharmacology: Official Publication of the American College of Neuropsychopharmacology*, Nature Publishing Group, Jan. 2017, www.ncbi.nlm.nih.gov/pubmed/27319972.

Dispenza, Joe. *You Are the Placebo: Making Your Mind Matter.* Hay House, Inc., 2015.

Doty, James R. *Into the Magic Shop: A Neurosurgeons Quest to Discover the Mysteries of the Brain and the Secrets of the Heart.* Avery, an Imprint of Penguin Random House, 2017.

Doty, James. "Hacking Your Brain for Happiness." TEDx Sacramento. Online video. YouTube. YouTube, 5 April 2016. Web. 20 October 2019

"Dr. Herbert Benson's Relaxation Response." *Psychology Today*, Sussex Publishers, www.psychologytoday.com/us/blog/heart-and-soul-healing/201303/dr-herbert-benson-s-relaxation-response.